Medicomarketing Writing

A Career for Health Science Students

Medicomarketing Writing
A Career for Health Science Students

Vishwanatha Matad

M. Pharm

Director, Medeka Health Private Limited,
Bengaluru.

Anusuya Dharman

M. Pharm

Consultant - Medical writer, Tulip Medcom,
Bengaluru.

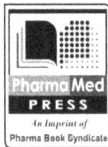

PharmaMed Press

An imprint of Pharma Book Syndicate

A Unit of BSP Books Pvt. Ltd.

4-4-309/316, Giriraj Lane,
Sultan Bazar, Hyderabad - 500 095.

Medicomarketing Writing: *A Career for Health Science Students by*
Viswanatha Matad and Anusuya D

© 2016, *by Publisher*

Published by

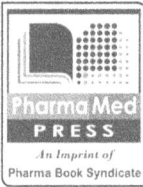

PharmaMed Press
An imprint of Pharma Book Syndicate

A Unit of BSP Books Pvt. Ltd.
4-4-309/316, Giriraj Lane, Sultan Bazar, Hyderabad - 500 095.
Phone: 040-23445605, 23445688; Fax: 91+40-23445611
E-mail: info@pharmamedpress.com

ISBN: 978-93-5230-104-1 (HB)

Preface

I have worked as a medical writer and later as a manager, recruiting, training, and overseeing the work of other medical writers. I wrote this book with an objective to provide an overview of medical writing as a fulltime profession, in particular, medicomarketing writing. This book would definitely help novice medical writers comprehend the responsibilities they may have at various levels: writing, project management, proposal writing (for medicomarketing only), recruiting, training, and retaining medical writers. It also provides an overview of the operations of medical communication companies, which would be helpful for product managers and medical advisors.

I started my career as a medical writer without any professional help from within the company or otherwise. I learnt the art of writing on trial and error basis. My friend and I have worked in this field for more than a decade, during which time we were working in the same or different organizations. This book reflects our collective experience in the medicomarketing business.

Viswanatha Matad

Director Medeka Health Pvt. Ltd.

Contents

Part I: Introduction

Part II: Writing Process

Part III: Variety of Medicomarketing Projects

Part IV: Writing Different Types of Articles

Part V: Biostatistics for Medical Writers

Part VI: Beyond Writing

43. Writer's Block   189

44. Performance Appraisal   192

PART - I

Introduction

Medical writers play a crucial role, not only in the process of drug development but also during the post-launch period. Being a successful medical writer involves understanding the product life cycle of the drug and having a practical approach towards the development of content for all stages of product life cycle. Success also depends on the personal attitude towards work, effective managerial skills, and the ability to train.

Chapter - 1

Medical Writing

S cientific writing began with the documentation of inventions and publication of theories way back from when man began exploring the laws of nature. This has left behind a legacy of the achievements of several scientists and researchers. Traditionally, scientific writing was limited to researchers, scientists or experts, who had to publish their research (academic writings/publications) for the documentation of their work, recognition, and the mutual benefit of fellow-researchers. Medical writing is scientific writing restricted to the profession of medicine. It is an integral part of the drug development process (right from pharmacological and preclinical/nonclinical studies to Phases I–IV studies), wherein a variety of documents are written based on the target audience. Background research papers are written for researchers involved in drug development. Protocol and regulatory writings are mandatory requirements for getting approval and conducting clinical trials. Original research writing is done based on the clinical trials. Subsequently, other documents are written in support of sales and marketing of the drugs developed. Writing for consumers/patient education literature is an extension of the sales and marketing strategies. In this context, medical writing has evolved as profession and medical writers play a key role in producing high-quality documents or articles for use across the drug development process.

1.1 Medical Writing Evolved as a Profession

Over the past decade, alongside the scientific and technological advancements, medical writing has evolved as a full time profession in the healthcare industry. Career opportunities in medical writing have provided an alternate career path to people specialized in medical and paramedical sciences, especially for those with a pharmacy background. A sudden bloom in this industry has left many of them clueless about the nature of the work, job responsibilities, and the career growth it offers. Despite the uncertainties, medical writing has evolved as profession owing to a number of reasons:

1. Not all researchers and doctors are good communicators, especially in written communication.
2. Writing is a time-consuming process. For many, time is too precious to be engaged in writing alone.
3. Inadequate or lack of communication of research would question the integrity of research done or the researcher himself. Moreover, miscommunication can lead to trial failures and re-trials, which have serious financial setbacks.
4. Journal publication houses are critical about language; poorly written articles would draw a bad reputation.
5. As such the data generated over years of research and experience is so vast that researchers/doctors themselves are unable to process and utilize it.
6. The majority of the publications are in English, which poses a problem to researchers from non-English speaking countries or to those who fail to adapt to the universal language, English.

1.2 Medical Writing Defined

Medical writing is an effective communication tool that helps translate scientific data into meaningful data, which can cater to the needs of target audiences viz., regulatory agencies, doctors, paramedics, pharmaceutical companies, and patients. According to the European Medical Writers Association (EMWA), "medical writing is about communicating clinical and scientific data and information to a range of audiences in a wide variety of different formats." According to the American Medical Writers Association, "medical communicators write, edit, or develop materials about medicine and health. They do this by gathering, organizing, interpreting, and presenting information in a manner appropriate for the target audience".

1.3 Medical Writing – Varieties

Medical writers are involved in preparing various documents during the course of the drug development process: clinical research, regulatory affairs, and sales and marketing (Figure 1.1). Pharmaceutical industries employ medical writers for writing regulatory as well as promotional or marketing-related documents. At times, owing to the diversity in writing, all these documents are not prepared in-house; pharmaceutical industries seek professional services from contract research organizations (CRO) and medicomarketing agencies.

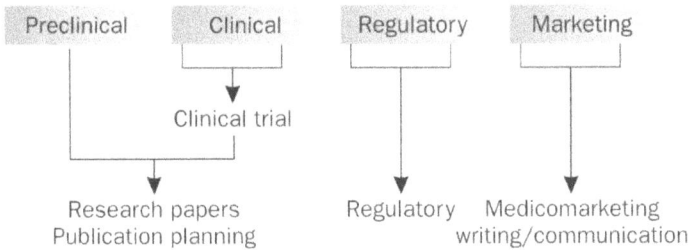

Figure 1.1: Medical writing involved in the corresponding stages of drug development

I would like to discuss only medicomarketing writing relevant to the Indian pharmaceutical industry; nevertheless, it is also worth mentioning that clinicians/academicians as well as pharmaceutical companies approach medical writers to ghost write primary/secondary (review) articles. Medical writers are acknowledged, given co-authorship or sometimes ignored. Medical writing associations are currently making an attempt to legalize ghost writing and give due credit to ghost writers.

The complete spectrum of writing right from drug development up to marketing is discussed briefly through Figure 1.2.

A

Target molecule identification and scrutiny

Screening vast data for potentially identifying target molecule

Reports submitted to researchers

B

Preclinical stage

Product development plans,
Animal study protocol,
Study report,
Toxicology report,

C

Clinical Phases I-III

Regulatory documents,
Investigator brochures,
protocols,
Informed consent documents.
Newsletter,
Analysis plans,
Safety reports,
Study reports (Phase I-Phase III), Developmental core safety information
Company core safety information
Data and safety monitoring board
Common technical document
Integrated summary of safety
Integrated summary of efficacy
Safety surveillance plan
Preapproval risk management plan

D

Regulatory

Investigational new drug application
Clinical trial authorization
Investigational device exemption
Pre-market approval

Contd...

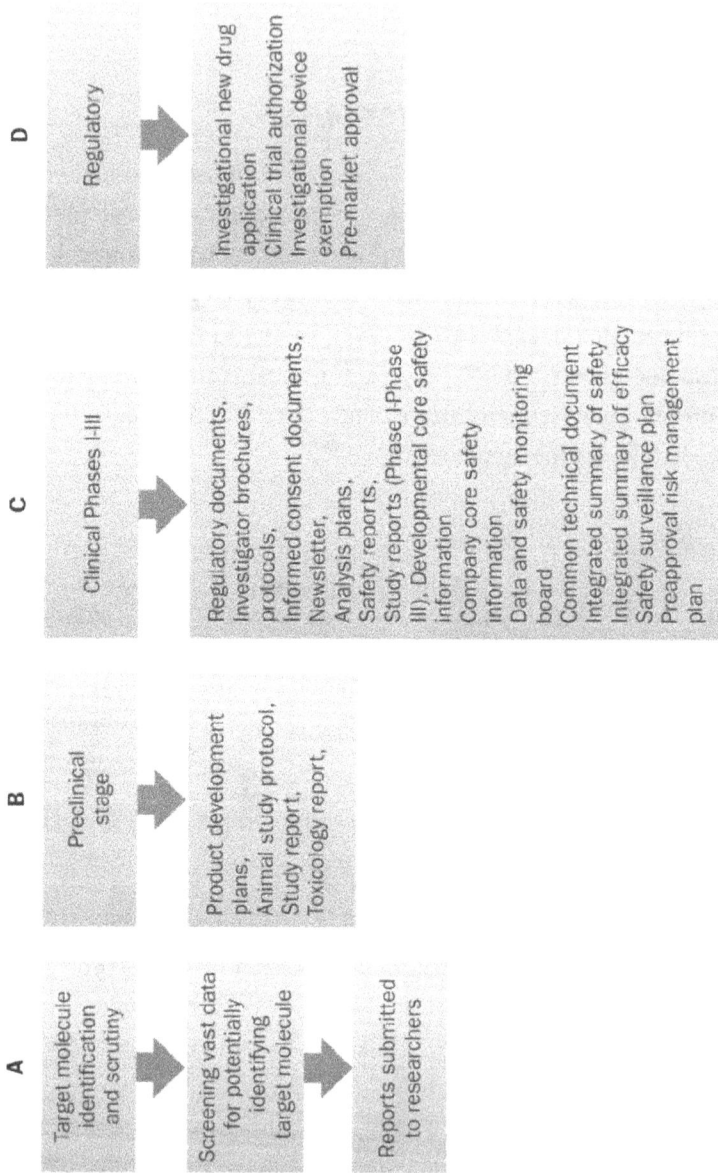

Figure 1.2: Complete spectrum of writing.

E

Phase VI
(Post-marketing)

Study report
Clinical safety report
Clinical expert report
Postapproval risk management
plan update plan
Safety narratives
Publication of scientific data

F

Medcomarketing

G

Product launch
(Scientific cum marketing inputs)

Product launch
(Scientific data only)

Submission dossier
Papers for publication
Literature reviews
Conference presentations
(with slides), abstracts
posters
Postconference highlights or
full proceedings

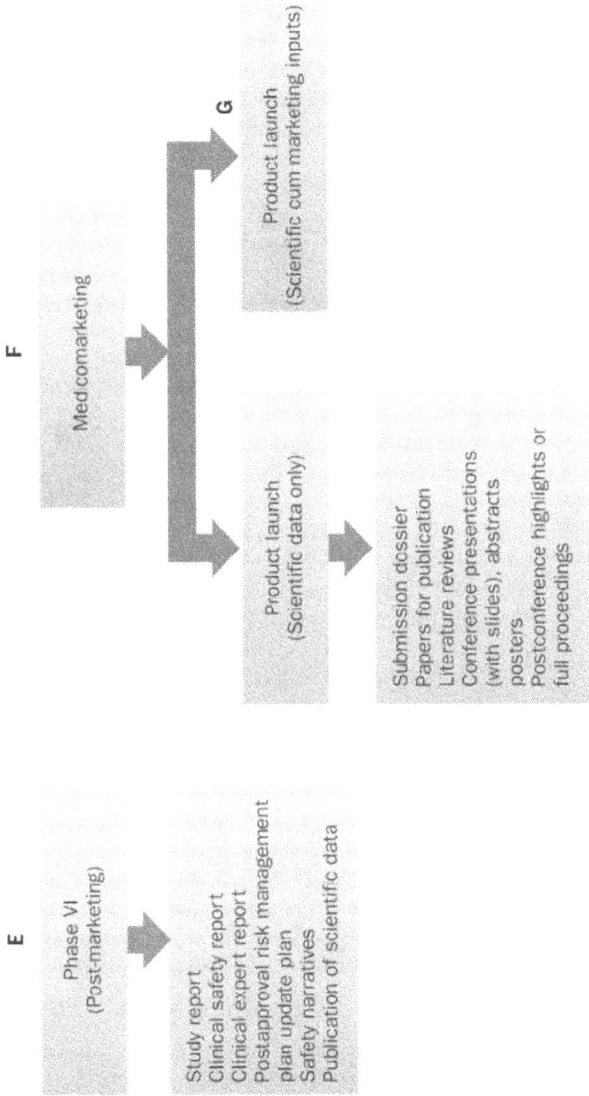

Figure 1.2: Complete spectrum of writing.

Contd...

G

Product launch
(Scientific cum marketing inputs)

For Product

Branding guidelines
Product monographs
Quality and assurance
documents
Strategic publication
planning/manuscripts

For Company

Product resource
documents
Staff work-shops
Internal newsletters
Competitor
assessments
Launch meetings

For Marketing

Product sales
materials
Slide kits
Advisory boards
Websites/multimedia
Key opinion leader
development
External newsletters

Congresses/events

Expert's meeting
Regional/global
meetings
Abstracts books
Commercial stands
Graphic displays
On-line quizzes
Handouts
Web-casts

**Public relations
(PR)/press release**

Media monitoring
PR manual
PR communiques
Core press
materials
Publicity campaigns
Press releases

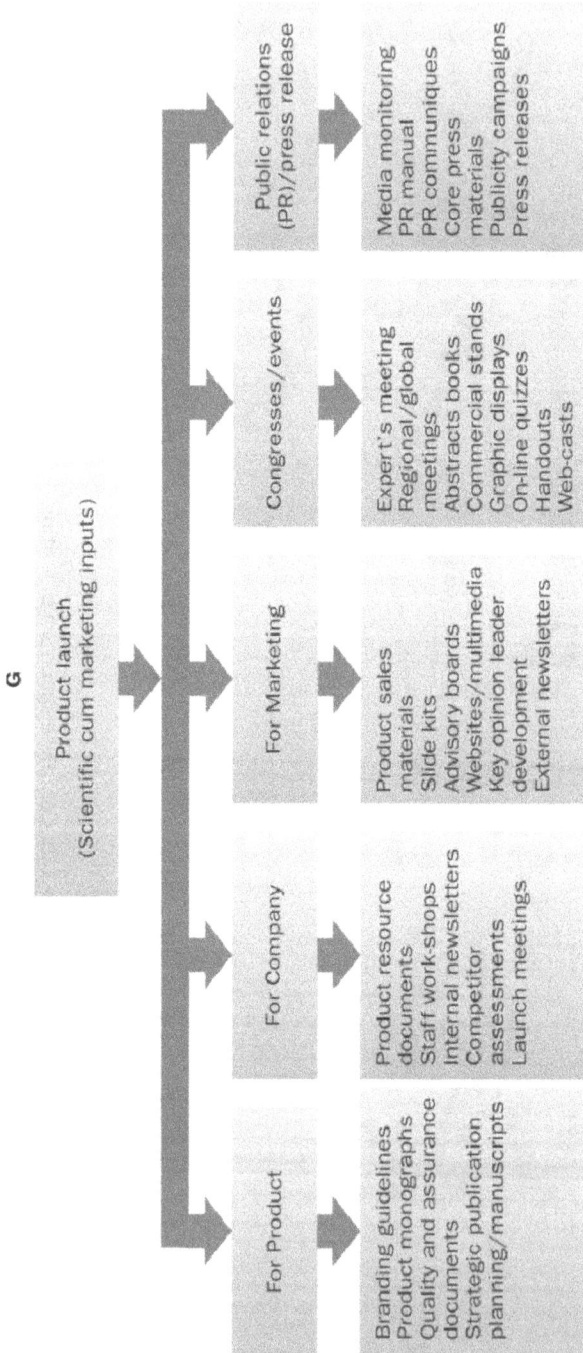

Figure 1.2: Complete spectrum of writing.

Chapter - 2

Medicomarketing Communication or Healthcare Communication

To sell pharmaceutical products, medical devices, and other healthcare products and services, doctors and/or patients must be made aware that the products and services are available. Providing scientific facts is an important ethical practice rendered by the industry to the medical community. Apart from providing literature related to the drugs that are marketed, as a goodwill gesture, pharmaceutical companies develop inputs for doctors, which serve as a value-add to their daily practice (diagnostic updates, guidelines, patient education materials, etc). Medical representatives use these different promotional materials as an excuse to meet doctors and indirectly accomplish the task of reminding the doctors of their company's brands.

In this context, a medical writer creates scientific marketing inputs that help the pharma marketing team to promote healthcare products or services. The promotional inputs developed serve many purposes:

- Provide information
- Engage doctors beyond the two minutes of the medical representative's meeting
- Persuade
- Remind
- For goodwill

2.1 Healthcare Information Needs of Physicians

"All physicians need to read medical literature regularly to stay up to date in their field," said Robert B Taylor. Doctors are eligible to practice medicine after completing their basic curriculum, but the information required during their day-to-

"All physicians need to read the medical literature regularly to stay up to date in their field"

day practice needs to be updated from time-to-time. Clinical practice is dynamic, with clinicians being challenged with complex problems in every stage of decision making, namely diagnosis, therapeutic choices, and implementation of clinical recommendations (Table 2.1). A practicing doctor can overcome these dilemmas by constantly updating oneself with the available information.

Physicians excelling in their profession largely attribute their success to practicing high-quality medicine. Moreover, the purpose of research is irrelevant until the information is transformed from 'bench to bedside'. Dissemination of data to clinicians is therefore important. On an average, experienced physicians use about two million pieces of information to manage their patients. Barring specialists, primary care physicians alone attend to more than 500 clinical topics in a year. Therefore, to practice high-quality medicine, doctors constantly seek to update their knowledge to manage their patients better.

Sources of information for clinicians to keep abreast with newer advances in medicine are diverse. However, the busy schedule of clinicians prevents them from setting aside qualitative time for assessing information from literature. On the other hand, searching for relevant data is by itself an art, which not many clinicians are adept at.

2.2 Sources of Information for Doctors

Various documents produced by researchers during the drug development process and beyond are too vast for a clinician to comprehend. Of late, physicians are encouraged to adopt and practice evidence-based medicine. Hence, doctors are obliged to acquire timely knowledge to ensure practice of high-quality medicine. Resources used by doctors in obtaining information include drug compendiums, colleagues, pharmacists, books, journals, information gateways [specialists or key opinion leaders (KOLs)], pharmaceutical representatives, and databases

Table 2.1: Information needs of clinicians

Practical need	Interest	Practical challenge
Diagnosis	Cause and interpretation of clinical findings	• What are the causes of the symptoms/physical findings? • Will a particular class of drug be effective for the given condition/symptoms?
Treatment		• What is the current recommendation for treating a particular disease/disorder? • Is any new drug introduced? • Does the drug have any new indications?
Adverse drug reactions	Drug prescription	• What is the black box warning issued by the regulatory bodies for a drug?
Diagnostic updates	Tests	• What are the latest diagnostic tools/tests available? • Which test is more reliable and cost-effective?
Epidemiology	Prevalence/incidence	• What is the trend in incidence of a particular disease or disorder? • Can the epidemiological findings of a particular disease or treatment outcome be extrapolated to other regions?
Knowledge updating	Nonclinical	• What is the latest information on the disease condition?

on the internet (Table 2.2). An article published in the BMJ in 1996 on the usefulness of information sources used by doctors seems appropriate even today (Table 2.3).

Table 2.2: Sources of information

Sources	Personal	Printed	Internet
Professional sources	Colleagues, KOLs, specialists, pharmacists, clinical pharmacologists, information centers	Journal articles, textbooks, drug formularies or directories	Databases, professional associations' programs, CMEs, interactive programs
Commercial sources	Medical representatives from the pharma industry	Journal articles, textbooks, drug formularies, advertising inputs	

Information gateways: By and large, clinicians look upon or consult 'educationally important physicians' or KOLs in the process of making clinical decisions. Doctors normally get to interact with KOLs during continuing medical education (CME) meetings or at conferences.

Journals: Practically, doctors cannot afford to subscribe to many journals. Even if journals are available through self-subscription or through other sources, their tight practicing schedules hinder them from acquiring knowledge. Moreover, seeking online practice-related information through journal scanning is tedious and requires skill in using appropriate keywords. More than 1700 medical journal articles are published every day. Lack of time, skill, and access to knowledge impedes doctors from practicing evidence-based medicine.

Drug directories: Drug directories provide list of brands available, indications, contraindications, special precautions, side effects, and cost of the product. Drug directories serve as prescribing clinical reference for practitioners. In addition, it also provides the contact details of manufacturers and distributors.

Databases: MEDLINE, EMBASE, and Cochrane Library are extensive electronic databases that are good sources of information. Again, the main constraint here would be the time and skill required to search these databases.

Table 2.3: Usefulness of information sources commonly used by doctors

Information source	Relevance	Strength of source	Usefulness
Standard textbooks	Good	Good	Most relevant
Evidence-based, regularly updated textbooks	Good	Good	Most relevant
Drug reference books	Good	Good	Most relevant
Journal clubs, Evidence-based medicine	Good	Good	Most relevant
Standard journal reviews/ Systematic journal review	Good	Good	Most relevant
Journal articles	Moderate	Good	Moderately relevant
Free medical newspaper	Good	Moderate	Moderately relevant
Internet	Good	Good	Most relevant, but should use authentic web resources
Cochrane library	Good	Good	Most relevant
Online searching	Moderate	Moderate	Moderate but depends on the skill of the physician to get appropriate data from authentic sources
Continuing medical education—lectures	Good	Good	Most relevant
Consensus statements	Moderate	Low	Moderately relevant
Colleagues or key opinion leaders (KOL)	Good	Relative	Most relevant
Clinical guidelines	Good	Good	Most relevant
Drug company representatives	Good	Good	Relevant but limited to the promoting brand

Annual meetings and conferences: Societies and organizational annual meetings do provide a platform for the exchange of practice tips and developments in medicine. Besides, these meetings are used to develop networking. However, these events usually happen annually, which does not provide enough time for doctors to discuss all the developments that may have happened in 365 days. At times, pharmaceutical industries play a pivotal role in organizing conferences and inviting guest lecturers. These meetings are truly informative, but are usually limited to KOLs and other renowned doctors. Logistic issues also prevent doctors from attending these meetings and conferences.

Literatures provided by pharmaceutical companies: Pharmaceutical companies as a part of their marketing strategy, offer promotional scientific materials to doctors. The different promotional scientific materials include visual aids, leave behind literature (LBL), booklets, product monographs, newsletters, etc. More than 75% of the doctors get most updates and recent advances from such literature distributed by pharmaceutical companies.

Doctors will not prescribe a new drug unless they have knowledge of its indications, advantages/disadvantages over older drugs, dosage, etc. Therefore, it is mandatory for pharmaceutical companies to furnish all this information, which turns out to be the main source of information for doctors. Doctors would not prescribe a drug, until they are sure of its usefulness for a particular disease or condition. Although, it is a common perception that promotional literature is biased, one has to acknowledge the scientific evidence that supports the claims made by the pharmaceutical industry.

2.3 Dawn of the Medicomarketing Writing Industry

Pharmaceutical companies are actively investing in generating vital information for doctors. Initially, product managers in co-ordination with the medical team developed all the promotional materials in-house. Later, they began to outsource the development of promotional material. Over a span of 10 years, realizing the market potential, many medicomarketing communication companies have evolved. There are many reasons for shifting from in-house development to outsourcing.

Efficiency: Observing the general trend in the pharmaceutical marketing strategy, it is obvious that timely development of qualitative scientific promotional inputs is critical. Product managers, as such, have different priorities and writing for scientific promotional inputs is usually not their top priority. The marketing division of many companies (including multinationals) lack core competency in developing the marketing inputs.

Number of brands: It is practically impossible to have independent divisions for handling all the brands of a company. The manpower required to generate promotional materials is enormous and cannot be afforded by all the companies.

Tug-of-war: There is always a difference in opinion between the product/brand managers and the in-house medical team over the scientific content of promotional materials. In this situation, it is practically an arduous task to get the inputs ready on time. To avoid any confrontations and delay, product managers began to outsource the content and medical advisors were required to oversee the content and give their approval.

Independent third-party: By and large, it is generally assumed that inputs developed by in-house pharmaceutical companies are biased. To overcome this obstacle or misconception, independent medical communication companies with good reputation are the best alternate to develop promotional material.

Writing is an art: Above all, writing itself is an art and medicomarketing writing requires additional skill and perfection that is beyond the scope of product managers, for whom writing is not their forte or job requirement. Nevertheless, a company is weighed or valued on the quality of the promotional input.

One-stop shop: The variety of promotional inputs required created logistic and financial issues, mainly with respect to design and printing. Marketing teams had to additionally deal with the purchase department, which further contributed to delays. Medical communication companies helped bring an end to such difficulties, providing pharmaceutical companies with a smooth and steady flow of promotional input.

Chapter - 3

Product Life Cycle and Various Promotional Inputs

Like any other product, medicines/drugs/diagnostics follow the typical product life cycle that is defined relative to time and sales. The life cycle refers to the period from before the launch of a product into the market until its final withdrawal. It is split into various stages. Scientific inputs are developed as part of the promotional input depending on the various stages of the product life cycle (Table 3.1 and Figure 3.1).

3.1 Pre-launch Phase

Marketing of drug begins well ahead from the time of its development or conception. Beginning early gives the product an edge. Typically, the pharmaceutical industry follows a publication plan, which begins as early as the preclinical stages of drug development. Early-stage market research provides direction and decision support. The various medicomarketing promotional inputs/strategies developed in the pre-launch phase include:

Teaser campaign: A strategy to sensitize the consumers/doctors/patients on target issues, highlighting a gap in therapy, creating a sense of urgency and need. The purpose of writing a teaser campaign is to invoke curiosity and prime the market before launching the new drug.

Advisory board: Advisory groups are groups of experts in a field, who convene meetings to discuss the product positioning anticipating the market/clinical needs and the outcome in clinical trials (phase II and III). In the advisory board meeting, experts usually form groups and debate over the pros and cons of the drug and its competitor (if any). The clinical expertise of various experts will provide valuable insight to identify the unique selling potential (USP) of the drug. Medical writers play a crucial role in documenting and translating the proceedings of the advisory board meetings for the internal purpose of the marketing department.

Table 3.1: Promotional inputs at different stages of the product life cycle.

Stages of product life cycle	Purpose	Promotional strategies
Pre-launch	Sensitize market or create awareness	• Teaser campaigns • Advisory board events • Training kits for medical representatives • CME kits for doctors • Complimentary journal articles • Detailing aids • Posters (patient education) • Product monographs
Launch	Brand building to capture the top notch place in the market	• KOL meetings/conferences/events • Complimentary journal articles • Publishing journal supplements • Booklets and treatment guidelines
Growth	Foster interest and promote loyalty	• Journals • Newsletters
Maturity	Target prescribers	• Brochures • Patient education
Decline	Revitalization, refresh, and repackage	• Detail aids • Newsletters • Clinical trial highlights

CME: Continuing medical education; KOL: Key opinion leader

Training kits: Medical representatives need to be trained about the new drug to be launched so that they can convey the right information to the doctors. Training kits for medical representatives, usually, are power point slides with speaker notes and a ready reckoner.

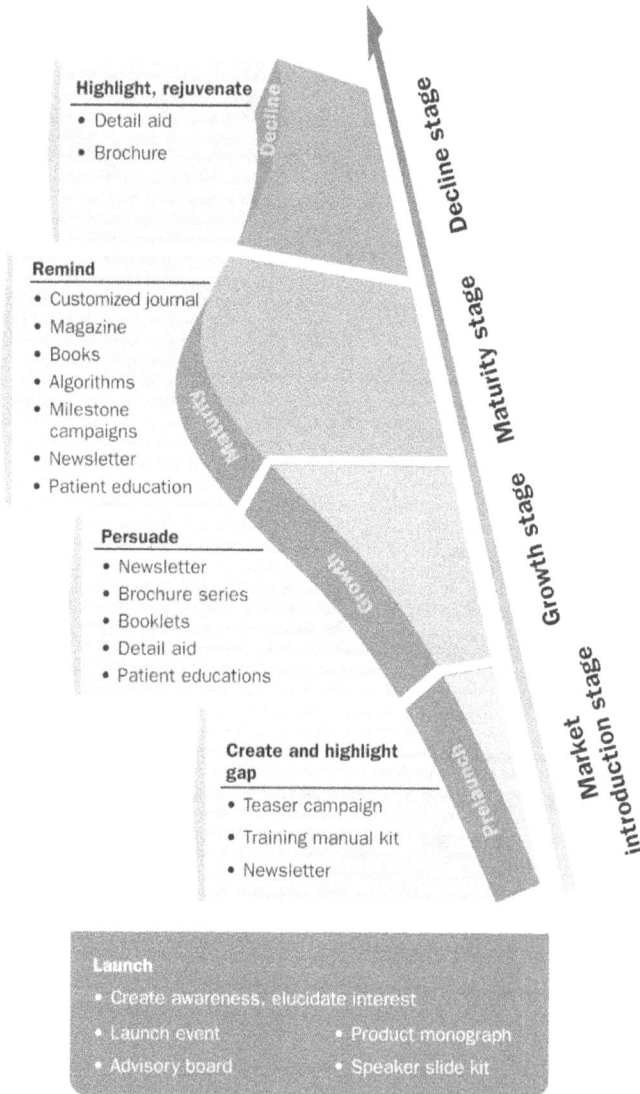

Figure 3.1: Medicomarketing communications throughout product life cycle.

Comparison chart: The USP of the launch molecule will be compared with that of the competitors to highlight the advantages.

Newsletter: A newsletter related to the product to be launched is circulated among doctors/paramedics. The topics written need not be directly related to the product, but they would be aimed at highlighting the gap in management and need for the new drug.

3.2 During the Launch

A successful launch is the key to long-term product sustainability. After thorough planning, the product launch usually begins with events/KOL meetings, wherein a number of inputs are required by the pharmaceutical companies:

- Invitations
- Programme and abstract booklets
- Highlights bulletin
- Workshop summaries
- Proceedings
- Video/DVD
- Detail aid
- Dosage card
- Clinical papers
- Monograph
- Newsletters
- Slide kits
- Testimonials
- Advertorials

3.3 Growth Phase

During the growth phase, doctors try out the new drug and if they are satisfied with the treatment outcome from their patients, they would continue to prescribe the medication. This would increase the sales of the new brand. During this juncture, medical representatives would require inputs to reinforce the advantages and the USP of the molecule. At this stage, based on the marketing strategies, different inputs are developed:

- Newsletters
- Brochures
- Booklets on USP
- CME kits
- KOL event proceedings

- Conference updates
- Case compendium

3.4 Peak/Maturity Phase

At the peak of the product life cycle, competitors would or would not have entered the market, but doctors would need to be reminded about the brand. At this phase, medical representatives require inputs to meet the doctor. The various inputs developed include:

- Newsletters
- Brochures
- Booklets on disease management
- CME kits
- KOL event proceedings
- Conference updates
- Patient education materials
- Case compendium

3.5 Decline Phase

The sale of a drug is likely to be affected by competition from other newer brands or new molecules. At this stage again, we need to reiterate the USP of the brand and highlight its advantages over the new molecules/brands. Usually in this phase, pharmaceutical companies seek to expand the market with new indications or diverse patient populations. The various inputs at this stage include:

- Newsletters
- KOL events proceedings
- Brochures
- Conference updates
- Booklets on USP
- Case compendium
- CME kits

3.6 Overview of Communication Plan

A typical plan for brand promotion using scientific communication is given in Tables 3.2 and 3.3.

Table 3.2: Scientific communication plan for a brand targeting healthcare professionals.

Program for healthcare professionals	Year 2012					Year 2013						
	Aug	Sep	Oct	Nov	Dec	Jan	Feb	Mar	Apr	May	Jun	Jul
Advisory board												
Journal articles												
Clinical symposia												
Advertising												
Sponsored educational column												
Newsletter												
Treatment guide												
Web Site												

Table 3.3: Communication plan for a brand targeting patients/consumers.

Programs for Patients/ consumers	Year 2012					Year 2013						
	Aug	Sep	Oct	Nov	Dec	Jan	Feb	Mar	Apr	May	Jun	Jul
Patient Educational Leaflets												
Public Health Talk												
TV program												
Radio program												
Doctors' Q &A												
Luncheon Talk												
On-going media Publicity												
Media workshop/ press Conference/ update												
Newsletter												

Chapter - 4

Qualifications and Skills

Qualification is not a major limitation in medical writing. Medical communication companies usually employ candidates with M Pharm, MBBS, MD, MSc (life science/biotechnology), BVSc, Phd in life sciences, BAMS/BHMS/journalism, BDS, and MDS. Some medical writers have a background in language studies and journalism. Ability and aptitude to understand medicine is the most essential skill required. Most companies prefer doctors and M Pharm graduates because of their thorough knowledge in pharmacology. Moreover, training these candidates is less cumbersome and more productive. In my experience, except for a couple of doctors, the medical writers whom I consider as good are M Pharm!

The skills required to be a good medical writer are discussed below (see also Figure 4.1).

Interest in reading and writing: Reading and writing go hand in hand. To be a good writer, you should be a good reader.

Passion: People with passion for writing only can enjoy this profession of medical writing and excel in their job.

Unfortunately, for many of them, it is a stop-gap arrangement, whose career destiny/pathway lies elsewhere.

Desired skills
- *Thirst for knowledge*
- *Understand the needs of both the client and the reader*
- *Search literature effectively*
- *Think critically*
- *Analyze and interpret data*
- *Simplify complex concepts*
- *Detail-oriented*
- *Well organized*
- *Deadline-oriented and flexible*
- *Able to work independently and in a team*
- *Accept criticism*

Interpersonal skills	Print and design knowledge	Self-motivated & independent worker	Good language skills
Good reader and writer			Practical and audience oriented
Passion for medical writing	Desired qualities of a medical writer		Comprehensive presentation
Curiosity with quick adaptability	Creativity and innovation	Willingness to travel (optional)	Accuracy and completeness/ perfectionist

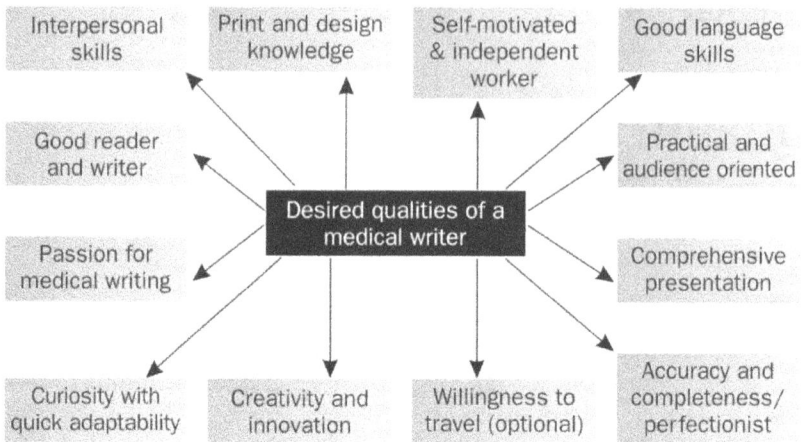

Figure 4.1: Desired qualities of a medical writer.

Curious: As a medicomarketing writer, you will be writing for different clients on different subjects, everyday. None of us can be experts in all specialties. Therefore you must be curious to learn and understand different subjects quickly.

Creative and innovative: Pharma industry is very competitive. Every client always wants 'something different', which would stand out among the many marketing inputs. I have heard clients complaining 'Kuch maza nahiaaya', despite giving good content. Creativity in medical writing can be inherent or acquired over a period of time. Creativity means presenting new and complex scientific data into simple data/language/graphical representation/tables. Moreover, imagination and creativity are necessary to develop various promotional inputs.

Creativity and innovation goes hand-in-hand. Innovation in medical writing is easily understood by those who know the pharmaceutical industry. Clinical trials/data available may be the same but it can be written and presented in different styles. Sometimes, you have to work on 2–3 projects related to the same drug/topics for different clients. Creativity and innovation in medical writing is synonymous to "filling the old wine in a new bottle".

Independent: Medical writers have to work independently. Medical writing *per se* is not a team work. The task of finding references, understanding, and paraphrasing/writing cannot be done by different people. As a medical writer, you must be able to comprehend all the available information and sometimes present controversial information in a fair and balanced way, which requires independent judgment. Timelines for the completion of projects are usually tight. Therefore, you should be able to organize your work independently and make decisions on your own depending on the situation.

Self-motivation: One has to be self-motivated to complete the projects within tight timelines. Despite writing good articles, client feedback can sometimes be demotivating. You would have to address all the queries of the client and yet be motivated to continue work. Medical writing is a kind of service industry, where client satisfaction is of utmost important. Remember—"The client is always right".

Practical and audience-oriented: A medical writer should be as practical as possible, because pharmaceutical companies cater to the needs of many across the medical community and patients. You must understand their audience and deliver work with the available financial resources. You should know and understand the purpose of various promotional materials, such as an article, an advertisement, video, press release, etc.

Perfectionist/detail-oriented/accurate: Every mistake is multiplied in thousands! (One mistake gets replicated in the all the print copies). The clients may have approved the final content but you are responsible for any mistakes that may arise in the final print. Mistakes not only have serious financial implications but also create bad reputation, which is not desired by the client and the medicomarketing agency. Therefore all important data has to be critically reviewed and interpreted accurately.

Good public relationship and managerial skills: Good public relationship and management skill will help in coordinating with other team members within the company, KOLs, and clients. In this context, good verbal and written communication skill is mandatory. Understanding the psyche of the client is important to sustain business.

Willingness to travel: Medical writers may need to travel to cover conferences/symposia or to conduct a key opinion leader (KOL) interview. You should be ready to travel, although it is not an essential requirement. Based on your personal interest, you can volunteer to attend and cover conferences

Computer skills: Computer versatility is advantageous as it increases your productivity. Besides a basic computer knowledge in Word, Excel, and PowerPoint, moderate-to-good typing speed is also desired.

Print and design-related aspects: You need not have a degree in printing technology, but you should have a fair idea about design and print jargons (which you can acquire over a period of time in the industry). Usually, the aesthetics of design is based on the therapeutic specialties, target audiences, type of input, and brand colors.

Chapter - 5

Career Path

Medical writing as a full time profession is a new age career; many fresh graduates who come for interview ask the questions, "What future can I have in medical writing? What is its growth potential?"

Growth in career is usually measured by position (designation/power) or salary (remuneration). In my opinion, intellectual growth is also as a parameter for career growth. Intellectual growth is the opportunity to learn new things related to writing, to do new things, and have new ideas continuously within the job. I (and some of my friends in this industry) regard intellectual growth more important than growth in terms of position or salary. There is no end to learning. Medical writing career is one of the best jobs to quench your thirst for knowledge, without much effort, because of the nature of the job itself. No additional time is required to keep oneself abreast with the latest developments in medicine. In fact, intellectual growth might not be rewarding in terms of money, but in this profession, it would help writers excel. Companies also should provide an environment for intellectual growth. Employees stimulated by interesting work and the ability to continue building their skills are more likely to be satisfied and remain with the organization for a longer time. It would help to have a more stable workforce and enhance the company's bottom line.

5.1 Employers

Medical writers are employed by:

- Medical communications companies
- Clinical research organizations (CRO)
- Pharmaceutical and biotechnology companies
- Medical books and journal publishers

- Advertising agencies
- Medical associations
- Health information technology companies
- Medical instruments and device companies

5.2 Career Ladder in a Medical Communication Company

Starting as trainee medical writer, you can scale-up to be a medical writer, team leader, editorial head, and so on (Figure 5.1). Almost all medical writers eventually move into management as team leaders (managing people and projects). However, if managing other people is not interesting to you, you can continue to be a writer. Most medical writers who started their career more or less a decade ago have scaled-up to be editorial heads. It is pretty easy to scale-up the management ladder in this career. If you have the right direction and the right attitude, it is possible to lead a team within a span of 1-2 years. There is a demand for efficient medical writers in this industry. At all stages of your career, you can continue to write, in addition to your other job responsibilities. Moreover, it is easy to recognize writers and their capabilities within a short span of time. Being a "small world", recognition as a good medical

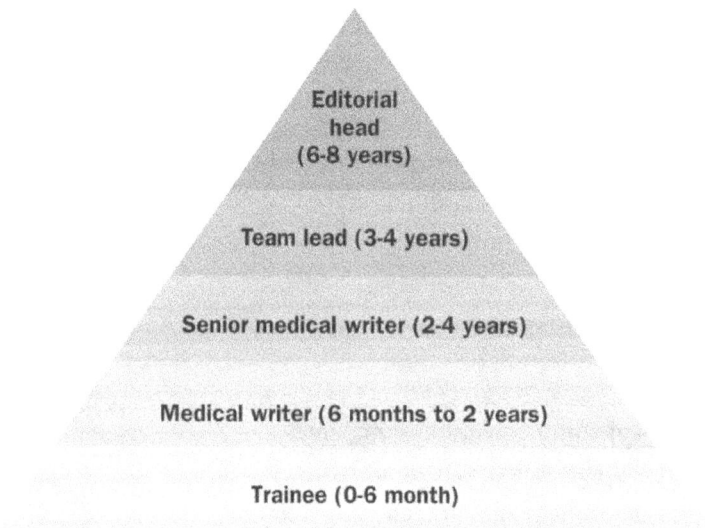

Editorial
head
(6-8 years)

Team lead (3-4 years)

Senior medical writer (2-4 years)

Medical writer (6 months to 2 years)

Trainee (0-6 month)

Figure 5.1: Career ladder in a medical communication company.

writer comes very easily and if talented, it is acknowledged. A medical writer with managerial qualities and better understanding of the business can even head a medical communications company. Some medical writers have set up their own companies. The best part of this career is that after a few years of experience, it is easy for you to become a freelancer, which also is a very lucrative option.

The designations used for different levels vary between companies, but the roles and responsibilities are more or less the same (Figure 5.2).

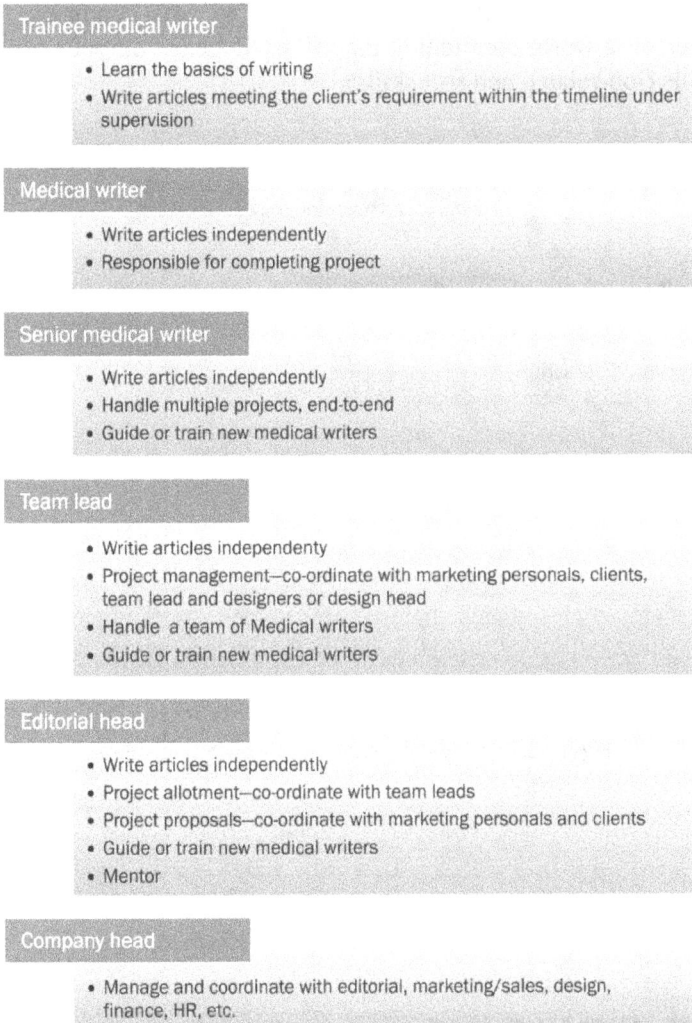

Trainee medical writer
- Learn the basics of writing
- Write articles meeting the client's requirement within the timeline under supervision

Medical writer
- Write articles independently
- Responsible for completing project

Senior medical writer
- Write articles independently
- Handle multiple projects, end-to-end
- Guide or train new medical writers

Team lead
- Writie articles independenty
- Project management—co-ordinate with marketing personals, clients, team lead and designers or design head
- Handle a team of Medical writers
- Guide or train new medical writers

Editorial head
- Write articles independently
- Project allotment—co-ordinate with team leads
- Project proposals—co-ordinate with marketing personals and clients
- Guide or train new medical writers
- Mentor

Company head
- Manage and coordinate with editorial, marketing/sales, design, finance, HR, etc.

Figure 5.2: Roles and responsibilities at different levels of the career.

5.3 Salary

Medical writing is lucrative even for a fresher who begins his/her career as a trainee medical writer. At present (2013), the usual starting salary for a fresher starts from 12,000 to 18,000. You can expect 10-25% increment every year depending on your and the company's performance. Evaluation of performance is easy and rewarding for good medical writers. Approximate salary range (in 2013) for the senior positions is given in the Figure 5.3. In fact, the salary for editorial head is even higher, with some companies even ready to offer company shares. However, it is worth mentioning that salary depends on your experience and skills (job-related and soft skills).

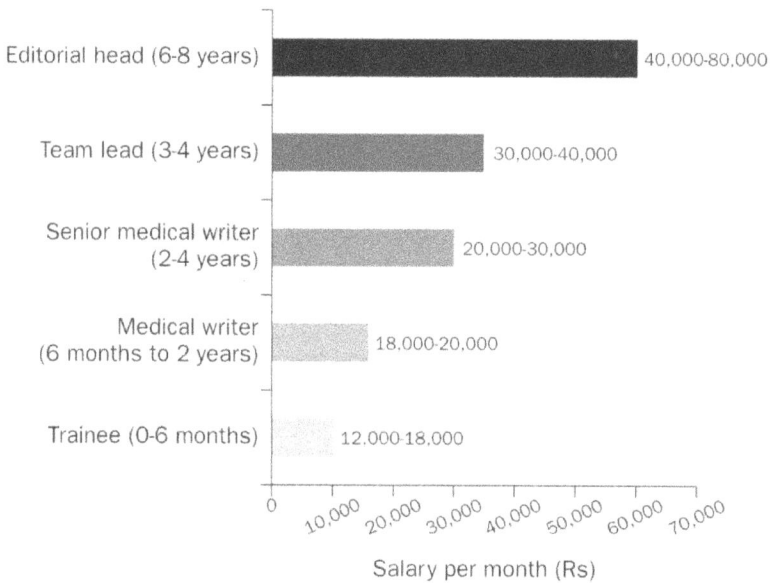

Editorial head (6-8 years) 40,000-80,000

Team lead (3-4 years) 30,000-40,000

Senior medical writer (2-4 years) 20,000-30,000

Medical writer (6 months to 2 years) 18,000-20,000

Trainee (0-6 months) 12,000-18,000

Salary per month (Rs)

Figure 5.3: Medical writer career path and salary.

Chapter - 6

Medical Communications: A New Age Growing Business

M edical writing catering to the Indian pharmaceutical medico-marketing department is flourishing. The total size of the Indian pharmaceutical industry was 55,454 crore (excluding exports and government purchases) in financial year 2009. Approximately, 10-15% of the sales turnover is spent for marketing/ promotional materials. This includes money spent on samples, gifts, conference sponsorships, medical literature/communication, advertisements in drug directories, etc. Of this, if we assume that 10% is spent on scientific literature/ communications, the market size of the medico marketing/medical

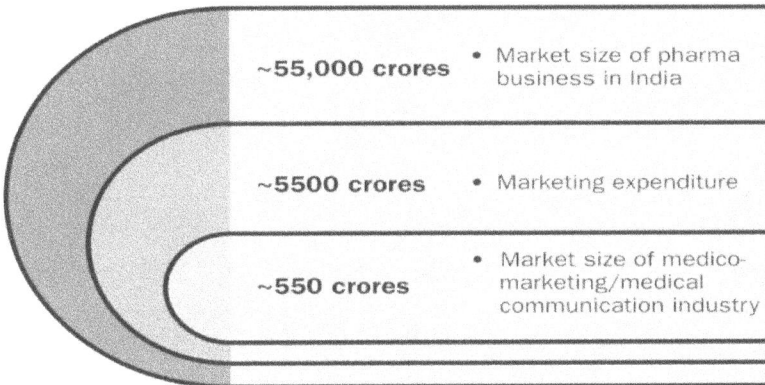

~55,000 crores	• Market size of pharma business in India
~5500 crores	• Marketing expenditure
~550 crores	• Market size of medico-marketing/medical communication industry

Figure 6.1: Market size of medicomarketing/medical communication industry (in 2009).

communication industry would be 554 crores (Figure 6.1). This business is fragmented among small/boutique design studios, advertising agencies, medical communication agencies, and in-house (development of promotional materials) and event management companies. Undeniably, on an average, the annual pharma industry growth has been at least 12%, which in turn assures a parallel growth for the medical communication industry as well as for the medical writer.

Chapter - 7

Where can you Learn Medical Writing?

Graduate or postgraduate pharmacy or medical courses does not offer course work on medical writing. There are no formally recognized courses offered by Indian universities. Some of foreign universities offer courses in medical writing but none specific to medicomarketing communication. Also, some courses in clinical research contain a module on medical writing. But those are related to clinical trials and are not useful for medicomarketing communications. All medical writers till date, have been trained in-house (medical communication company/pharmaceutical company) or have had "on-the-job" experience. You can learn by seeing, doing, and listening. Initially, we learnt medical writing by "on-the-job practical experience". Otherwise, if you are lucky, you could be trained by your seniors. Look up to your seniors and colleagues to learn. In fact, we decided to write this book to enable others like us to have a better insight into medicomarketing writing in India. Good medical writers, whom we know till date, have learnt the nuances of medical writing from "on-the-job" experience and through observation.

Workshops and seminars on medical writing are organized by various medical writers associations (American medical writers association, European medical writers association and such others). Based on the response this book receives, we may be encouraged to offer the right medical writing training for medicomarketing.

Chapter - 8

Finding a Job

In my opinion, medical writing is the best option for fresh graduates. My mentor used to say, "It is better to hire a fresher, with common sense". Within a couple of years of my medical writing career, I was given the responsibility of hiring medical writers! It was challenging, because I had no clue as to how to select candidates. I prefer postgraduates (preferably M Pharm) because I believe that their curriculum prepares them to work independently.

8.1 How to Search for Job?

Experienced candidates can find jobs through newspaper advertisements, college alumni, job consultants/placement services, internet, and social networking websites. Fresh graduates have to largely depend on their network of seniors and friends. I strongly advice fresh graduates to make a list of medical communication companies and then directly meet the human resource department to submit their resumes. Resume should be simple and free from grammatical and spelling errors. You have to follow-up with the human resource department on the status of the vacancy.

8.2 How to Give an Interview and Submit Your Assignments?

During an interview, I suggest that, besides answering the questions, make yourself clear as to what the job has to offer. Ask questions to know the way the industry works. Take a clue from the products that they are producing. You will be asked to write a test article to assess your writing ability and understanding of the subject. Your assignment will be assessed based on accuracy of information, references used, paraphrasing, grammar and spelling, content structure, and supporting tables and figures.

8.3 Pros and Cons of Medical Writing Jobs

Every job has its own advantages and disadvantages and medical writing is no exception.

8.3.1 Pros of Medical Writing

- Dynamic and intellectually rewarding.
- Constant exposure to new scientific/clinical information.
- Offers the satisfaction of deciphering science to target audience in an appropriate format.
- Demand for variety and creativity keeps oneself motivated.
- Mandatory project planning makes you well organized.
- Quick career growth.
- Interaction with other departments (design and copyediting) increases the scope for lateral learning.
- Opportunities to travel and attend seminars/conferences.
- Opportunities to meet key opinion leaders and interact with them.
- Apart from medical writing, you have the opportunity to improve and/or develop new business.
- Opportunities to learn from seniors and mentor novice medical writers.
- The need for medical writers will NEVER DIE. Pharma industries will ALWAYS need good medical writers to sustain their business. We can proudly say, "The pen is mightier than the sword".
- Increased need for medical writers makes the skill marketable.
- With a couple of years of experience, one has the liberty to work as a consultant or freelancer from home.
- It is the best job for women and for men looking for a desk job.

8.3.2 Cons of Medical Writing

- Tight deadlines might turn out to be stressful, because timelines are important in this industry.

- At times, one will be forced to write on a limited choice of therapy area. You may have to repeatedly write on the same topic for different clients.

- Comprehending vast data is tiring and you may not get enough time to understand the subject.

- Alien or complex subjects may need to be learnt within a limited time.

- Client satisfaction is of utmost importance —"the client is always right" and this may be depressing or demotivating at times.

- Despite tight deadlines, there is an immense pressure on writers to deliver QUALITY within minimum time.

- Multitasking is inevitable. You will be forced to handle multiple ongoing projects without drastically compromising on the timelines of other projects.

- Medical writers are prone to occupational hazard of desk work. You would have to be constantly at a desk, looking into a computer monitor.

- Projects are individual responsibilities and therefore, you might end-up working during vacations or holidays.

Chapter - 9

Typical Project Flow in Medicomarketing

The typical project flow can be understood from the figure 9.1. The process is more or less the same, with slight deviations from one company to another. An average turnaround time is usually 45–60 days from the time of project initiation. Based on the project, the editorial head/team lead/editors would interact with the client.

- Initially, the client, usually the product managers, would get in touch with the marketing personal of the medico-marketing company and explain his requirements.
- The marketing team will pass on the client requirement to the editorial head.
- The editorial head will check for the project feasibility and then make a proposal and forward it to the marketing team.
- The marketing team will add the project cost and forward it to the client.
- The client after reviewing the proposal will accept with or without changes and confirm the project.
- The project is confirmed by the marketing team after booking the purchase order.

Marketing sends the clients' final project brief to the editorial head. The project brief in addition to the confirmed topics will have specifications related to the size of the product (A4, 1/4th demy, 1/6th demy, tabloid), print color (single, two, four), preferred colour according to clients preference/product, any specific photos/images to be used, logo of products, and companies (if any), any special message on the cover page, number of pages, header (if required), etc.

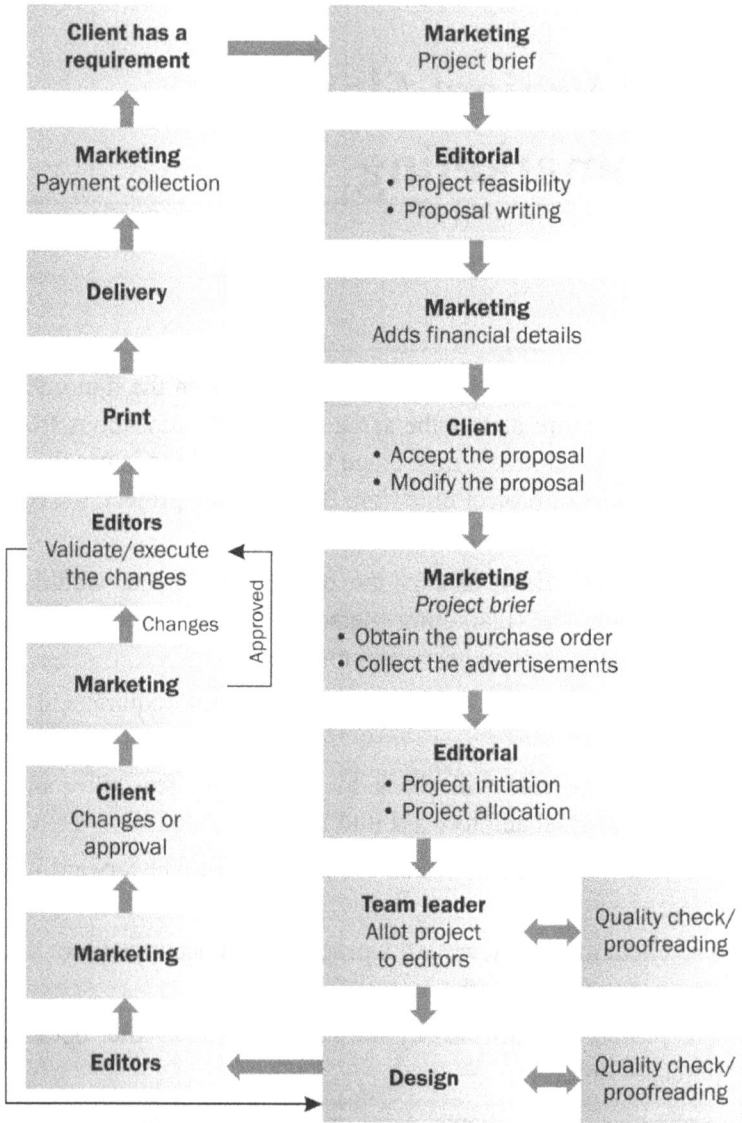

Figure 9.1: Typical project flow in medicomarketing industry.

- The editorial head will allot the project to a team leader.
- Team leader allots the work to editors.
- Editors will search data, collect references and write the articles.
- The articles are sent for proof reading, relevant changes are done by the editors and forwarded to design.
- Designers would format the content according to the project specifications. After quality check, they would forward it to editors.
- Editors will forward the literature to marketing, who in turn would send it to the client.
- The client would review it and if necessary will take the approval from their medical advisors.
- The client might or might not ask for changes.
- The final literature would be sent to print and delivered to the client.
- Realization of the payment can be expected within 45-60 days from the time of delivery.

PART - II

Writing Process

The writing process begins with identifying a topic to write, which is usually the toughest hurdle for a writer. But in medicomarketing writing, you do not have to worry about the topic. Topics are decided by the pharmaceutical companies based on their marketing strategy. Writing appears to be a single step process but it involves many distinct stages.

- Understanding the topic/brief/client requirement
- Resourcing
- Understanding/reading
- Writing content approach or outline
- Writing the article

Chapter - 10

Understanding the Topic/Brief/Client Requirement

D o not start writing without understanding the purpose of the article/topic that is assigned to you. First and foremost you need to consider:

- Client's need
- Readers (target audience)
- Format of the output

10.1   Client's Need

From here on, the pharma industry will be referred to as 'the client' as the context is related to the immediate product manager, who communicates the pharma industry's needs to us. The purpose of the product (customized scientific content)/project may be to inform, persuade, or entertain. You need to ask a lot of questions to understand the client's need:

1. Which is the generic and what are its indications?
2. What are the unique selling properties (USP)?
3. Who is the target audience?
4. What does the client want to derive?
5. When and how will the scientific content be used?
6. What is the deadline?

Subsequent to the preliminary background work and the client's requirement, I have observed that logically all the thought processes involved in understanding the client's brief revolve around the following criteria:

- Stage of the generic in the product cycle
- Stage of the brand in the brand life cycle
- Benefits of the generic or USP of the drug vs. competitor's drug
- Target indication
- Target audience

These criteria are self-explanatory, but to help you understand better, we will explain with examples. Before we start discussing each criterion in understanding the brief, I would like to highlight on two aspects.

1. ***Drug name vs. brand name:*** For the sake of convenience, a generic drug refers to the drug's name. The brand refers to the brand of drugs that are marketed by the pharma companies.

2. ***Generic vs. brand life cycle:*** Generic life cycle refers to the product life cycle of the innovator brand. Brand life cycle is the product life cycle of various subsequent brands that are introduced in the market. Hence, generic and brand life cycles are dealt separately because they are different. All brands do not have the same product life cycle as that of a generic.

Generic vs. brand life cycle

Example 1: AstraZeneca, first launched Meronem (meropenem) in 2003, and the product life cycle for Meronem brand and the generic meropenem were the same. In 2004, other companies launched meropenem. At this juncture, the generic (meropenem) and the brand (Meronem of AstraZeneca) were in the growth phase, while Zaxter (the brand of Alkem) was in its introductory phase. Hence, the marketing inputs for Alkem and AstraZeneca on the same generic will vary. Alkem required visual aids, monographs, newsletters, and brochures. On the other hand, AstraZeneca needed inputs focused on the latest updates and was looking to expand the indications for the drug.

10.1.1 Stage of the Generic in the Product Cycle

The marketing strategy of client will depend on the stage of the generic in its product life cycle. Another way to understand the brief is to know the stage of the product in its market life cycle. Recollect the product life cycle graph (introduction, growth, maturity and decline) discussed earlier.

Stage of the generic in the product cycle

> **Example 1:** In 2003, meropenem, both generic and brand (Meronem by AstraZeneca), was in the launch phase.

> **Example 2:** Few molecules such as esomeprazole, telmisartan, and atorvastatin were all in the growth phase in 2011, wherein the inputs required by them varied.

> **Example 3:** Tranexamic acid tablet was introduced in the early 1960's for hemorrhage or risk of hemorrhage in those with increased fibrinolysis. Recently, tranexamic acid was relaunched as an injection formulation. The tablet formulation was already in the decline stage, but with the introduction of the injection, tranexamic acid (Cyklokapron injection by Pfizer was introduced in 2010) was revived.

Proposal for stage of the Generic in the Product Cycle

> **Example 1:** AstraZeneca's Meronem (meropenem): Annual plan for meropenem comprising of visual aids, monographs, and series of newsletters for different indications and target audiences:

1st year
- Comparison charts for medical representatives (MR)
  - Vs. 3rd generation cephalosporins (4 or 5 different molecules) so that MRs know the differences and highlight the advantages
- Product monographs (during launch)
- Detail aids
  - Nosocomial pneumonia
  - Intra-abdominal infections
  - Meningitis
  - Sepsis
- Booklets covering safety and efficacy of meropenem in different indications
  - Meropenem in nosocomial infections
  - Meropenem in intra-abdominal infections
  - Meropenem in meningitis
  - Meropenem in sepsis

2nd year
- Brochures
  - Meropenem vs. imipenem
  - Management of pseudomonas infections

- Conference coverage
  - IAIM—Indian Academy for Infection Management
    - Campaign before the meeting
    - Electronic version of the meeting
  - Dr. Shaw's talk on de-escalation therapy
    - Newsletter and CD of conference
- Newsletters series "Critical care updates" 8 issues (quarterly for 2 years)
  - Meropenem in sepsis
  - Meropenem in nosocomial pneumonia
  - Meropenem in febrile neutropenia
  - Meropenem in intra-abdominal infections
  - De-escalation therapy
  - ESBL resistance
  - Selective digestive decontamination
- Case studies

10.1.2 Stage of the Brand in the Brand Life Cycle

Once the brand is launched, it passes through the three phases of brand life span, namely, growth, peak and decline. Based on which stage the brand is in, the marketing input strategy will vary.

Stage of the Brand in the Brand Life Cycle

Example 1: In India, MSN launched a new generation antiplatelet drug, prasugrel (Prasusafe) in 2010. For promoting this molecule, the client wanted numerous inputs. Visual aids, monographs, and subsequently a series of newsletters were developed.

Example 2: Nexium (esomeprazole), which was launched in 2005, was in the maintenance phase in 2011. In 2011, AstraZeneca began promoting Nexium to cardiologists and otolaryngologists for low dose aspirin-related upper gastrointestinal disorders and laryngopharyngeal reflux, respectively. The indication of the drug (proton pump inhibition) was extended to different populations.

Example 3: Metoprolol (launched in 1992) is a cardioselective beta-blocker used in the management of hypertension and has been in the market for more than 30 years. Metoprolol was obviously in its decline phase. IPCA began promoting metoprolol XL/CR in combination with amlodipine. Atenolol, the age old cardioselective beta-blocker is commonly prescribed by general physicians. IPCA targeted against atenolol and promoted metoprolol XL/CR subtly as a combination using a series of brochures and newsletters.

10.1.3 Benefits of a Generic or USP of the Drug vs. Competitor Drug

Every generic comes with advantages and disadvantages. Depending on the stage of the brand and the research updates on the molecule, the clients prepare various inputs. Usually, comparisons are drawn against the competitor molecule belonging to the same class or different class.

Benefits of a generic or USP of the drug vs. competitor drug

Example 1: At the time of launch of prasugrel (2010) by MSN, clopidogrel was the standard drug. The limitations of clopidogrel were: modest antiplatelet activity, significant inter individual variability, hyporesponsiveness, and delayed onset of action. The USP of prasugrel was more potent antiplatelet activity, faster onset of action, and less interpatient variability. The theme for the series of newsletters was based on each disadvantage of clopidogrel and advantage of prasugrel.

Example 2: Alkem was promoting pantoprazole, the proton pump inhibitor (PPI) for acid-related gastrointestinal disorders. Pantoprazole is a PPI that effectively inhibits gastric acid secretion in adults, adolescents, and children. Comparisons of the various PPIs in pharmacodynamic and pharmacokinetic studies have demonstrated only minor differences of questionable clinical significance. The main differences associated with pantoprazole are its irreversible and specific proton pump binding leading to greater bioavailability and longer duration of action than other PPIs. In addition, pantoprazole is more stable in neutral to moderately acidic conditions than omeprazole, lansoprazole, or rabeprazole, suggesting a lower propensity to become activated in slightly acidic body compartments. To date, no drug-drug interactions have occurred with pantoprazole, which is an important consideration for elderly patients, who often need to take several drugs. A series of brochures were developed to highlight the advantages of pantoprazole over other PPIs.

10.1.4   Target Indication

Usually, the approved indications are the primary indications, which are broad. For example, NSAIDS are indicated for management of pain, which includes tooth pain, headache, muscular pain, spasms, etc. Nevertheless, based on the available clinical evidence, the pharmaceutical industries promote the drug across various subgroup populations (elderly patients, patients with comorbid conditions, pre- or postmenopausal women, etc).

Target Indication

Example 1: Let us consider the drug telmisartan. Telmisartan is officially indicated for the treatment of hypertension and cardiovascular (CV) risk reduction in patients, who are intolerant to angiotensin converting enzyme (ACE) inhibitors. Hypertension includes mild, moderate, severe, and uncontrolled hypertension. Hypertension is present in patients with diabetes, renal failure, metabolic syndrome and other comorbid conditions. Hypertension management is recommended for primary or secondary prevention of coronary artery disease (CAD). Hypertension is also observed in pregnant women and children. Therefore, telmisartan can be promoted for mild, moderate, severe or uncontrolled hypertension based on the subgroup of population. Depending on the marketing strategy of the client, telmisartan can be promoted for cardiologists, diabetologists, general practitioners, or consulting physicians. A series of brochures can be developed on the following topics to position telmisartan in the following subgroup population

- Telmisartan for mild-to-moderate hypertension
- Telmisartan for hypertension in people with diabetes
- Telmisartan for hypertension in people with chronic kidney disease
- Telmisartan for hypertension in people with metabolic syndrome
- Telmisartan for hypertension in people with dyslipidemia
- Telmisartan for primary prevention of CAD
- Telmisartan for secondary prevention of CAD
  - o   Stable angina
  - o   Unstable angina or non–ST-elevation myocardial infarction (MI)
  - o   ST-elevation MI
  - o   Left ventricular (LV) dysfunction

10.1.5 Target Audience

An indication of the drug permits its use across multiple specialties. Depending on the clients' marketing strategy, the target audience for promotion of the drug varies.

Target audience

> **Example 1:** Mefenamic acid is an NSAID indicated for the management of pain. One company would promote mefenamic acid to pediatricians, while another company would promote it to gynecologists.

> **Example 2:** One company would promote atorvastatin to general practitioners (GPs) for primary prevention, while another company would promote the same statin to cardiologists or interventional cardiologists and consulting physicians for secondary prevention.

> **Example 3:** Tranexamic acid is promoted to
> - Urologists: Role of tranexamic acid in prostate surgery
> - Gastroenterologists: Role of tranexamic acid in gastrointestinal bleeding
> - Surgical oncology: Role of tranexamic acid in oncosurgery
> - Surgeons: Role of tranexamic acid in liver transplant surgery

10.2   Readers

Readers may be doctors (GPs, consultants, specialists, super specialists, super-super specialists), medical representatives, patients, consumers, nurses, or pharmacists. You need to write according to their basic level of knowledge. Put yourself in the shoes of the audience. Ask yourself questions about the reader:

1. What can I expect them to know?
2. How do they read?
3. What is the information that is needed or interests them?

Readers may be annoyed if you use unusual words and complex sentences. You would be overestimating their knowledge. If you write laboriously about obvious things, you are underestimating their knowledge. You must learn to strike a balance to avoid either overestimating or underestimating their knowledge.

You should also know how they read. Most doctors do not read from cover to cover (or A to Z). They usually browse through the contents and read only important or highlighted points. There are too many journals and literature to read in-depth. So, doctors glance through the articles in their free time between consultations. Therefore, it is better to write succinctly and use figures, tables, and highlighting points to grasp their attention on gist of the article. If there is lot of text (verbose), they may not even pick up the article. Doctors seek information to fill gaps in their knowledge related to their daily practice.

10.3 Format of the Output

Think about the final product before writing. Usually the client chooses the format of the desired output. The format can be 4 to 6 page newsletters, 2 to 6 page brochures, 8 to 100 page booklets, slidekits (power point presentation in CDs and booklet) for doctors or medical representatives, KOL interviews in CD format or executive summaries in booklets/brochures. For example, the complications of diabetes can be made into a 100-page booklet or a 4-page brochure. You can also write storyboards for a patient education film. The style of writing and amount of text should depend on the number of pages and the size of the paper.

Chapter - 11

Resourcing
___

Medical writers are not fiction writers. You need to have references to support every sentence you write. Finding the references is not a single path that proceeds straight from initial question to final answer. It is actually more like a cycle. Initial questions lead to a few references, which lead to more references and more questions, and so on.

11.1 Information Sources

References can come from two sources:

1. Libraries.

   (a) Printed books, journals, magazines, dictionaries

2. Internet

   (a) Search engines

   (b) Medical search engines

   (c) Databases

   (d) Websites of journal publishing companies

   (e) Government websites

   (f) Journal websites

   (g) Pharmaceutical company corporate websites

   (h) Brand websites (patient-oriented and healthcare professional oriented)

   (i) Specialty websites sponsored by pharmaceutical companies

   (j) Medical news websites

(k) Medical and nonmedical image websites

(l) Medical college/University websites

(m) Medical CME websites

(n) Medical library websites

Before the 1990's, writers had to run from library to library, rack to rack, in search of references using bibliography journals. Now with the internet, references can be searched and resourced at the click of a mouse. The internet is a great tool for research, but finding quality material and using them to your advantage can be challenging.

11.1.1 Search Engines

A search engine is a tool used to locate web pages according to specific keywords. Some writers endlessly search for the "better article" using a search engine. Nevertheless, you should know where to start and when to stop. There are many search engines.

- Google
- Yahoo
- Altavista
- Bingo
- Lycos

You can use any search engine. But you should be familiar with the advanced search options available and type of results you get. I like Google as a default search engine as it gives me what I want.

Search engines return with results from wide varieties of websites. You need to evaluate the websites before considering them as references. Books and journal articles generally go through a long process of fact-checking, editing, and revising before being published. Nevertheless, anyone with a computer and internet access can post any information on the web. Just because the information is published online, it does not mean it is true or reliable. Some web sites change frequently and sometimes disappear quickly. Evaluate the website while browsing to make resourcing efficient and effective. Consider only authentic sources of information for writing your article. The best way to evaluate a website is to ask yourself a list of questions.

1. Who is the creator of the site?
2. What is the purpose of the site?
3. Who is the audience of this site?
4. Is the site affiliated to a business or university?
5. Does the site offer idiosyncratic information about a particular disease or therapy?

Some information in the web address itself will give you a clue about the type of web page you are viewing. A non-profit organization is indicated by 'org'. Government branches are indicated by '.gov'. Business sites are usually indicated by '.com' or '.net'. Educational institutions are indicated by '.edu'. Official United States' sites are indicated by '.us'. Sites published in the British Isles are designated '.uk', while '.au' indicates Australian sites.

After you identify the type of website you are viewing, you must assess it for credibility, which, however, is difficult to ascertain. Information posed on the website depends in large part on the author; unfortunately, the author's name may not be clearly listed on the web site. Sometimes, the author's name may be listed, but his/her credentials may not be provided. In such cases, it is always better to check with your senior writers or team leads whose experience would help you decide on the credibility of the data from the website.

11.1.2 Databases

Databases contain information that has been screened for its quality by the application of standards that typically ensure a high level of validity and clinical relevance. Databases should be your first choice for resourcing data. Although there are many databases, by default, I begin with 'pubmed' as most of the peer-reviewed journals are indexed here. Once I collect the list of references and abstracts, I will either go to the journal website or to publisher's website to get the full text, if required. I would search other databases only if there are no references or few references in pubmed. For India-specific information, I prefer the 'IndMED' database. The following are the most common health- and medical-oriented evidence-based databases.

11.1.3 Pubmed/Medline

MEDLINE (Medical Literature, Analysis, and Retrieval System Online) database is the premier source for bibliographic and abstract coverage of biomedical literature. Developed by the U.S. National Library of Medicine (NLM), MEDLINE includes information from Index Medicus, Index to Dental Literature, and the International Nursing Index, in addition to other sources in the areas of allied health. Pubmed contains more than 16 million records from more than 4,600 journals indexed. Approximately 75% of the records provide abstracts.

You can limit article searches by:

- Type of article [clinical trial, review (systemic or narrative review), editorial, letter, meta-analysis, guideline.
- Field (title, author, keyword, abstract, entire article)
- Age (infants, adults, elderly)
- Date (old-new)
- Publication date (from 1966-till date)
- Gender
- Language
- Humans or animals
- Subset (AIDS, cancer, dental, etc).

When I start searching, I use keywords in "title" as the limit. This option gives me an idea about the minimum number of articles available on the topic with the keywords in the title. When I need only clinical studies related to a drug, I use "clinical trial" as a limit. "Review articles" and "Full text articles" options are useful to access only review articles and full texts. Another useful option is "Related article" available with every reference. There are several other useful features:

- The Journals Database lets you look up journal names, MEDLINE abbreviations, or ISSN numbers.
- Single Citation Matcher allows you to verify or source a single citation.
- The Batch Citation Matcher allows you to verify multiple citations,

- A Clinical Queries form is available for a user to search for the therapy, diagnosis, etiology, and prognosis of a topic.
- My NCBI is a stored search feature that allows users to store and automatically update searches.

11.1.4 Excerpta Medica (EMBase)

EMBase contains more than 20 million records from more than 7,000 active authoritative journals, including over 1,800 titles that are not in MEDLINE. It is maintained by Elsevier Science. It contains journals related to human medicine (both clinical and basic biological research, experimental) and selective coverage of: nursing, dentistry, veterinary science, psychology, and alternative medicine, including homeopathy. It can be accessed from **http://www.embase.com** and via authorized database vendors. However, it requires subscriptions. I do not use this regularly.

11.1.5 IndMED

IndMED is a bibliographic database of Indian biomedical journals **http://indmed.nic.in.** It is maintained by a center jointly setup by the NIC (National Informatics Center) and ICMR (Indian Council for Medical Research) to cater to the information needs of the Indian medical community. A subsection called medIND contains fulltext articles of 38 journals indexed in IndMED.

11.1.6 Psychinfo

Produced by the American Psychological Association, PsycINFO covers professional and academic literature on psychology and related disciplines, including medicine, psychiatry, nursing, sociology, education, pharmacology, physiology, linguistics, and other areas **(http://psycnet.apa.org)**. It includes references and abstracts from over 1300 journals (and dissertations) in more than 30 languages and book chapters and books in the English language. Over 50,000 references are added annually.

11.1.7 Ovid

Ovid, maintained by Wolter Kluwer, provides information for students, professionals and institutions in medicine, nursing, allied health, and pharmacy **(http://www.ovid.com)**. Ovid offers vast medical and scientific content via OvidSP and is published by the world's leading publishers. It houses:

- More than 3,000 ebooks, including 60 book collections and archive collections of critical historical material, publisher collections, and topical collections

- Over 1,200 premium, peer-reviewed journals plus 50 journal collections, including archive collections and packages based on publisher or subject

- Over 100 bibliographic and fulltext databases

11.1.8 TOXNET

The Division of Specialized Information Services of NLM created and maintains TOXNET® **(http://toxnet.nlm.nih.gov)**, a collection of toxicology and environmental health databases. TOXNET includes the Hazardous Substances Data Bank (HSDB®), a database of potentially hazardous chemicals, TOXLINE® (the world's toxicology literature), and ChemIDplus® (a chemical dictionary and structure database). The TOXLINE database **(http://toxnet.nlm.nih.gov/cgibin/sis/htmlgen? TOXLINE)** is the NLM bibliographic database for toxicology, a varied science encompassing many disciplines. TOXLINE records provide bibliographic information covering the biochemical, pharmacological, physiological, and toxicological effects of drugs and other chemicals. It contains over 4 million bibliographic citations, most with abstracts and/or indexing terms and CAS Registry Numbers. TOXLINE references are drawn from various sources organized into component subfiles which are searched together but which may be used to limit searches as well. TOXLINE covers much of the standard journal literature in toxicology, complemented with references from an assortment of specialized journals and other sources. I have used TOXNET to get comprehensive information on many generic drugs.

11.1.9 J-East

J-EAST is the largest free-of-charge searchable database of citations and abstracts of documents published in Japan in all the fields of science, technology, and medicine **(http://sciencelinks.jp/j-east/)**. J-EAST contains documents from about 3,000 sources, including academic publications, serials, proceedings, and technical reports of hospitals, universities, and enterprises published in Japan. Abstracts of articles in Japanese have been translated into English.

11.1.10 The Cochrane Database of Systematic Reviews

The Cochrane Database of Systematic Reviews is a database of regularly updated systematic reviews prepared by The Cochrane Collaboration. The reviews are presented in two types: 1. complete reviews and 2. protocols for reviews currently being prepared (the background, objectives and methods of reviews in preparation).

11.1.11 Hinari

Hinari is a World Health Organisation (WHO) sponsored free website for poor countries **(http://extranet.who.int/hinari/en/journals.php)**. HINARI Access to Research in Health Programme provides free or very low cost online access to the major journals in biomedical and related social sciences to local, not-for-profit institutions in developing countries. It includes major journals from major publishers including Blackwell, Elsevier Science, the Harcourt Worldwide STM Group, Wolters Kluwer International Health & Science, Springer Verlag, and John Wiley.

11.1.12 Websites of Publishing Companies

In all the following websites, access to abstracts would be free, but access to the full text article would need subscription or one time payments.

- ScienceDirect (http//www.sciencedirect.com/)
- Wiley Online Library (http//onlinelibrary.wiley.com/)
- Ingentaconnect (http//www.ingentaconnect.com/)
- Springer (http://www.springer.com/)
- Nature Publishing Group (http://www.nature.com/)

- Cambridge Journals Online (http://www.journals.cambridge.org/)
- Oxford University Press Journals (http://www.oxfordjournals.org/)
- Taylor & Francis (http://www.tandf.co.uk/journals/)
- Informa healthcare (http://informahealthcare.com/)
- Karger Medical and Scientific Publishers (http://www.karger.com)

11.1.13 Medical News Websites/Magazines

Some of the following websites exclusively present daily medical news. Certain magazines also present journal articles in the form of news. Such articles are easy to comprehend and provide up-to-date knowledge on the latest happenings in the world.

- Eurekalert
- BBC health
- MSN health
- Medscape
- Science daily
- The new scientists

11.2 Key Words and Boolean Search

After knowing where to search, you should know how to search. References are indexed using key words, words in the title, and words in the abstract. Using the 'right term' while searching is very important to get the right references from databases and search engines. The problem with looking for literal words is that there are usually lots of synonyms and variations for any word. MEDLINE includes a set of concept terms called MeSH (Medical Subject Heading). Use a MeSH rather than a title or abstract word, because all articles related to it would be indexed under that one term. The NLM has a book of all the MeSH terms.

You can also look up papers by author. This can be very helpful in tracking down a report mentioned in other sources where they usually give the name of the researcher, but no citation to the paper. If you find one interesting paper, you may want to use this feature to look up other papers by the same authors. MEDLINE allows the use of Boolean search options such as 'AND', 'OR', 'NOT', and 'NEAR', which can be used along with keywords. Using these terms would help narrow your search.

- **AND:** Requires both the terms to be are present anywhere in the article.

- **NEAR:** Both terms to be found within a certain number of words of each other.

- **OR:** Requires at least one of the terms to be present.

- **NOT:** Excludes any document containing the term.

Boolean search

> **Example 1:** If you use 'atorvastatin AND stroke', pubmed will give you articles containing 'atorvastatin' AND 'stroke'. If you use atorvastatin NOT stroke, it will give references on atorvastatin without the word 'stroke' anywhere in the article. For the search term 'atorvastatin OR simvastatin', pubmed will retrieve articles on both the drugs.

While using search engines use alternative terms or synonyms. You can also restrict the search by file type (pdf, ppt, video, etc). Confidence in employing the right keyword or Boolean search stems from common sense and fair knowledge about the subject. With the help of senior writers, you can empower your search with practice.

Chapter - 12

Reading and Understanding the References

Most of the reading will happen while resourcing itself. Reading and writing are very closely related. If you do not understand the article which you are writing about, chances are you would not be able to write the article very well. Do not start writing without understanding all the references you have collected. For better understanding your reading strategy must be logical and involve:

1. Skimming

2. Specific reading

3. Reading in depth

Skimming involves getting an overview of the contents available. Most of the skimming can happen while resourcing. While skimming:

- Look for a specific keyword

- Get a general idea without putting effort into close reading.

- Read the opening paragraph and the conclusion carefully.

- Read the first and last sentence of each remaining paragraph to get some idea of the main points.

- Look for phrases that act as sign posts to the main ideas or messages in the text, or that give clues to anything specific you might be looking for.

- Use a marker pen to mark out any items that you want to re-read, or to refer later.

You may skim through the article if you have already read the text thoroughly and want to recall the main points. While skimming, highlight important points and make notes in the margin. This will be useful to refer back at the time of writing. Segregate articles into clinical trials, review articles, etc. and according to the flow/outline of your article, so that it would be easy to refer back. Also identify the articles to be read in-depth.

In-depth reading is the most essential of all reading strategies. You need to read an article thoroughly in order to comprehend the ideas and arguments it contains. In-depth reading takes more time and you may need to read certain difficult sections more than once.

To understand the articles, you should be familiar with different types of medical journals, different types of articles appearing in the journals and research methodologies.

12.1 Type of Journals

1. **Broad-based peer-reviewed journals:** These journals carry articles related to any specialty. Four major journals in this categories include:

   (a) JAMA

   (b) BMJ

   (c) Lancet

   (d) NEJM

2. **Specialty-specific peer review journals:** Almost all associations of any specialty publish journals. Most of these journals carry original articles. Rarely, journals like the American Association of Family Physicians publish articles on disease management than original articles.

3. **Controlled circulation journals:** Such journals are published by medical publishing companies. Most of these journals do not contain original research articles. Examples include Consultant, and Practitioner.

12.2 Type of Articles Appearing in the Journals

The various types of articles that appear in a journal are:

1. Lead articles
2. Review articles
3. Meta-analysis
4. Editorial

5. Letter to editor
6. Short communication
7. Original research articles
8. Guidelines
9. Case reports/studies
10. Consensus Statements

12.2.1 Lead Articles

These articles would usually discuss contemporary research topics that are expected to see a breakthrough. These are the kind of articles that sensitize the readers to new breakthroughs in science.

12.2.2 Review Articles

Review articles are a summary of all the current work in a single area. Review articles can be simple or a systematic compilation of several trials in the same field. A simple review and systematic review is differentiated by the method used for compiling data. The purpose of a systematic literature review is to evaluate and interpret all available research evidence relevant to a particular question. Review articles are primarily intended to keep professionals updated on the latest research under one umbrella. Naturally, review articles contain a very extensive list of useful references. Review articles are one of the best places to begin your detailed search. Review articles help in providing an overview of the subject, but ensure that you read the latest review in order to not miss out on the latest data on diagnosis, treatment, or drugs/interventions.

12.2.3 Short Communication

Short communication is like an expert opinion that usually debates on the outcomes of the latest or landmark trials. The communication usually communicates the opinion of peers in that field, in the context of the clinical applicability of the data.

12.2.4 Editorial

An editorial is a short paper written by either the journal's editor(s) or by a guest editor that addresses an issue of interest to a given journal's readership. Editorials may introduce topics covered within a journal issue, present pros and/or cons, clarify positions, or provide readers with updated information on new methods or procedures.

12.2.5 Letters to Editor

A letter to the editor is usually a brief communication written in response to an article previously published in the journal. Some letters include extensive commentary with careful referencing to the literature and thus can serve as a valuable source to the primary research literature. The information is usually valuable to researchers in that field and clinicians who look for solutions to fill the gaps in therapy or diagnosis.

12.2.6 Meta-Analysis

Meta-analysis is a systematic, quantitative analysis (usually of published literature) that statistically analyzes the data of multiple studies with similar outcomes. They are used to increase the statistical power available to assess the effect of an intervention on key outcomes and to better understand the size of that effect, as well as to assess the outcome effect on subcohorts. The quantitative statistical analysis of many study results distinguishes a meta-analysis from a systematic review. Meta-analyses have considerable impact and are usually considered critical parameters in implementing changes in clinical practices and guidelines.

12.2.7 Primary/Original Research Articles

Primary studies report research, first-hand. These are based on the research results. Original research articles can be of different types depending on the method of research. These are discussed in a later part of the book. Original research articles have a quite a rigid format. They are usually demarcated as abstract, introduction, methods, results, discussion, and conclusion. This format is commonly referred to as IMRAD.

Abstracts provide a complete overview of the research: The study objective/background, the method, experimental population and intervention, results of the study in brief and study conclusion. Given the function of the abstract, you should read it first to get a general understanding about the whole paper/research. **Introduction** usually provides a brief review of previous research, a rationale or reason for the research and an outline of the study objective. The **Method** sections describe the trial design, patient population, intervention, and measure of outcome parameters employed in the research. The **Results** section describes the results found. You will sometimes find the results and discussion sections combined. The **Discussion** section provides an interpretation of what the results actually mean in terms of the field and the original research question or hypothesis. Read the discussion section to understand what the results mean. **Conclusion or General discussion** section details the implications of the research and make recommendations about further research or policy and practice in the relevant area. Read the conclusion or general discussion section for an understanding of the key issues resulting from the research.

12.2.8 Guidelines

A guideline (practice guideline; clinical practice guideline) is a systematically developed evidenced-based statements written to help practitioners make appropriate decisions in specific clinical circumstances. Good guidelines draw their conclusions from a careful review of primary studies, landmark trials, meta-analyses and systematic reviews.

12.2.9 Case Reports/Studies

A case study is a report of a single interesting or multiple 'unusual' clinical cases. These studies usually are an investigator's actual clinical encounters with patients. Clinicians publish case studies for providing insights in diagnosis or treatment to fellow clinicians in the same field.

12.2.10 Consensus Statements

Guidelines are usually evidence-based. In cases where adequate trials are not available, to facilitate clinical decisions, expert professionals/KOL in a specific field meet with an agenda and discuss the pros and cons of the proposed guidelines and arrive at a consensus via voting. Once a unanimous or major consensus is arrived, the guidelines are issued as consensus statements which are purely based on the clinical practices. It is intended to advance healthcare professionals' and/or public understanding of a targeted health problem, practice, or issue. Examples include the statement on Medical Nutrition Therapy in Diabetes Management by the American Diabetes Association and the Delphi Consensus on Management of Peptic Ulcer Bleeding by the American Gastroenterology Association.

12.3 Research Methodologies (Study Design)

To understand the references, you need to know various research methodologies used in original research articles or the review articles.

Identifying the type of the clinical study is important for understanding the strength of an article (Figure 12.1). The relevance and strength of the available data is based on the type of the study (Figure 12.2).

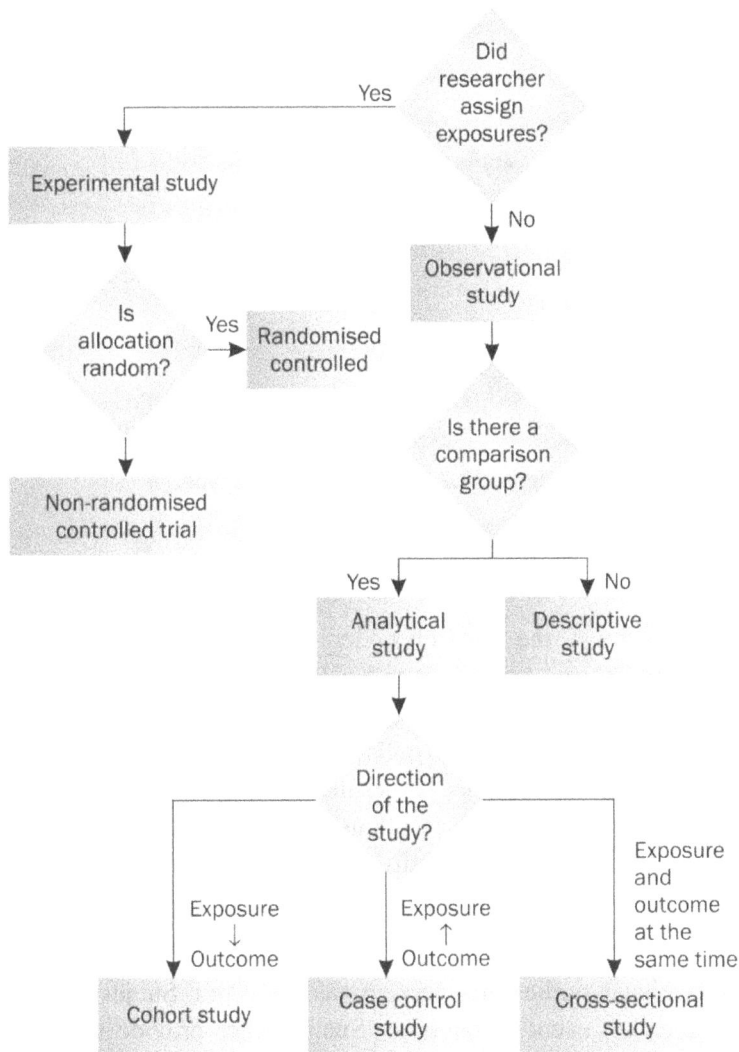

Figure 12.1: Study designs in clinical research.

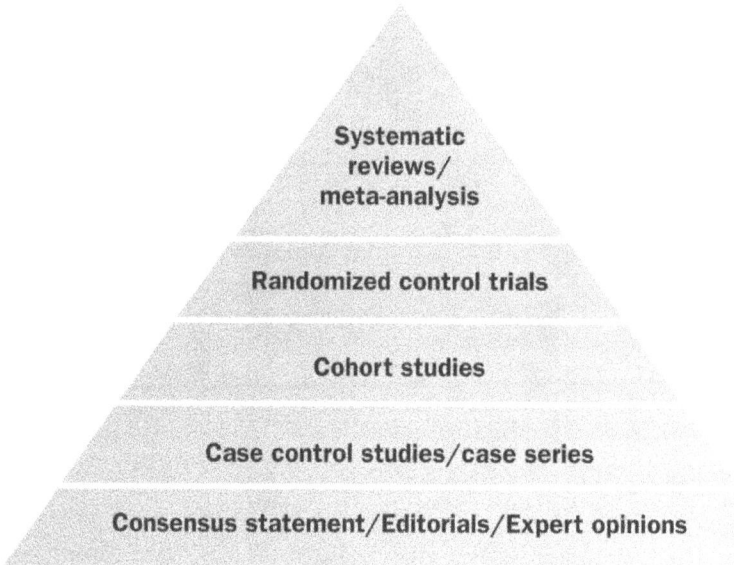

Figure 12.2: Strength of article type.

12.4   Research Classification

First and foremost, the research undertaken can be as simple as either 'observational' or 'experimental'. Parallel to literary meaning, 'observational' implies observing the patients or the condition and recording the data by merely collating data through observations and questions. On the other hand, 'experimental' means that the patients are subjected to experimental interventions and thereafter, the relevant data is recorded. Let us see each type individually, in brief.

12.4.1   Observational Studies

In observational studies no interventions are given. Subjects are merely observed for an event in question. Such studies provide estimates and examine associations of events in their natural settings without recourse to experimental intervention. Observational studies can be differentiated as descriptive or analytical (Table 12.1).

Table 12.1: Types of observational research

Descriptive	Analytical
Case reports	Ecological studies
Case series	Cross sectional studies, two group studies
Cross-sectional studies	Case-control studies
Longitudinal studies	Cohort studies

12.4.1.1 Descriptive Studies

Descriptive studies describe what is observed in patients.

1. **Case Reports:** Case reports are hardly considered research articles. They are descriptive studies on single individuals with unusual clinical presentation, which may or may not be treatable. Such case reports are published with an objective of sharing the physicians' experience (with respect to diagnosis or treatment) or seeking clinical answers with respect to diagnosis and treatment.

NCBI   Resources ⊙   How To ⊙

PubMed.gov   [PubMed ▾]
US National Library of Medicine
National Institutes of Health   Advanced

Display Settings: ⊙ Abstract   Send to: ⊙

West Indian Med J. 2012 Jun;61(3):302-4

A patient experiencing pseudoseizures: a case report.

Joseph F, Quinlan J.

University of Wollongong School of Medicine, Australia. David Berry Hospital, 85 Tannery Road, Berry, NSW 2535, Australia. john.quinlan@sesiahs.health.nsw.gov.au

Abstract
Pseudoseizures are a relatively complex problem of unknown aetiology and prognosis. They can at times resemble genuine seizure attacks but they have no abnormal electroencephalographic (EEG) activity. Understanding the patient's unique psychological background appears to be fundamental in managing seizure frequency. Pseudoseizures can be disruptive to a person's lifestyle, limiting their ability to function and progress in society particularly when it comes to employment or social interaction. The case discussed involves a 59-year-old man who presents with what is believed to be seizure-related activity but through the course of clinical evaluation, this turned out to be pseudoseizures.

PMID: 23155992 [PubMed - indexed for MEDLINE]

⊕ Publication Types, MeSH Terms

⊕ LinkOut - more resources

2. **Case Series:** A series of unusual clinical presentations (more cases than usual of a rare condition) is called as a case series.

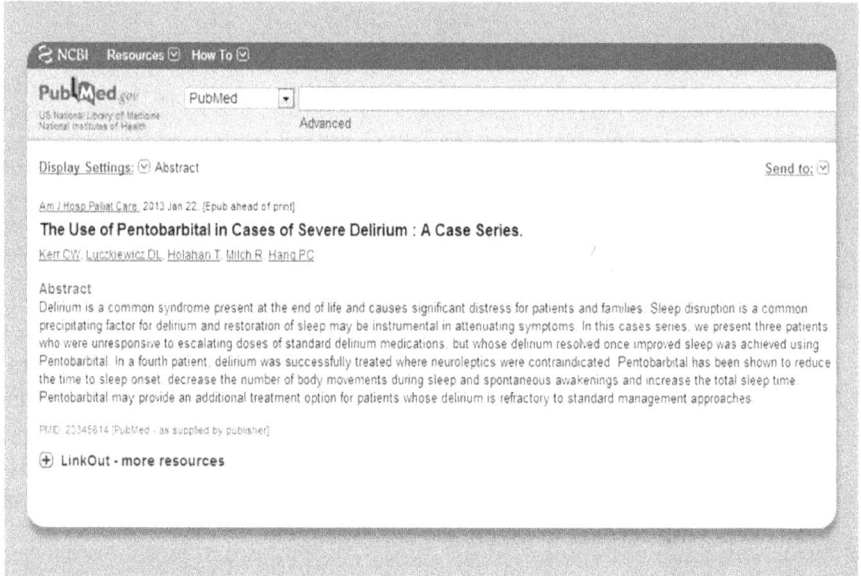

3. **Cross-sectional Studies:** A section of population is assessed for the presence or absence of any clinical feature in question. A prevalence study is a typical cross-sectional study. Prevalence studies report on the frequency of a disease or condition in a given population. The study design for cross-sectional study is depicted in Figure 12.3.

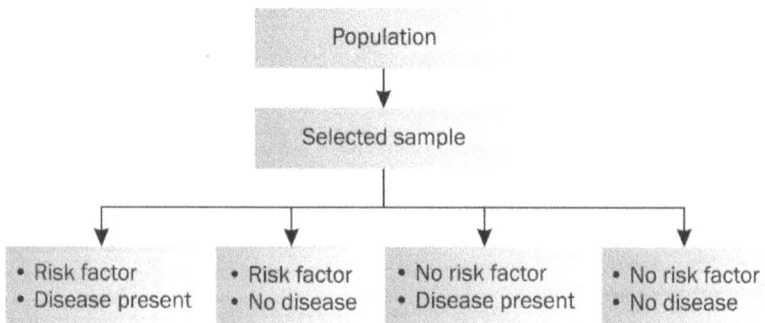

Figure 12.3: Study design for cross-sectional studies.

Display Settings: ⊙ Abstract   Send to: ⊙

Osteoporos Int. 2013 Jan 23 [Epub ahead of print]

Do patients with osteoporosis have an increased prevalence of periodontal disease? A cross-sectional study.

Marjanovic EJ, Southern HN, Coates P, Adams JE, Walsh T, Horner K, Devlin H

Arthritis Research UK Epidemiology Unit, Centre for Musculoskeletal Research Institute of Inflammation and Repair, The University of Manchester, Manchester, M13 9PT, UK. elizabeth.marjanovic@manchester.ac.uk

Abstract

The study examined if women with osteoporosis were at increased risk of periodontal disease. Three hundred eighty females aged 45-65 years with recent dual-energy X-ray absorptiometry (DXA) scans of the spine and proximal femur agreed to a dental examination. No association was established between the presence of severe periodontal disease and osteoporosis.

INTRODUCTION: The purpose of this study is to determine whether patients with osteoporosis have an increased severity and extent of periodontal disease, taking full account of confounding factors.

METHODS: Volunteer dentate women (45-65 years), who had undergone recent DXA of the femur and lumbar spine, received a clinical examination of their periodontal tissues by a single trained operator who was blind to the subject's osteoporosis status. Clinical examinations were performed within 6 months of the DXA. Basic Periodontal Examination score, gingival bleeding score, periodontal pocket depth, recession and calculus were the periodontal outcome measures. Potential confounding factors were recorded. Logistic regression was performed for the dichotomous outcome measure of severe periodontal disease (present or absent) with osteoporotic status, adjusting for confounding factors.

RESULTS: There were 380 dentate participants for whom DXA data were available. Of these, 98 had osteoporosis. When compared with osteoporotic subjects, those with normal bone mineral density were significantly younger (p = 0.01), had a higher body mass index (p = 0.03) and had more teeth (p = 0.01). The prevalence of severe periodontal disease in the sample was 39 %. The unadjusted odds ratio for the association between osteoporosis and severe periodontal disease was 1.21 (0.76 to 1.93). The adjusted odds ratio analysis including other covariates (age, smoking, hormone replacement therapy, alcohol) was 0.99 (0.61 to 1.61).

CONCLUSION: No association was established between the presence of severe periodontal disease and osteoporosis.

PMID: 23340945 [PubMed - as supplied by publisher]

⊕ LinkOut - more resources

4. **Longitudinal Studies:** In this study type, the subjects are followed-up on one or more occasions over a longer duration of time to determine their prognosis or outcome. Longitudinal studies show the incidence of a new disease or the prognosis of an existing disease in a predefined population (or at risk population) over a defined period of time.

Display Settings: ⊙ Abstract   Send to: ⊙

Soc Psychiatry Psychiatr Epidemiol. 2013 Feb 48(2):205-14. doi: 10.1007/s00127-012-0541-6. Epub 2012 Jul 3

Family cohesion and posttraumatic intrusion and avoidance among war veterans: a 20-year longitudinal study.

Zerach G, Solomon Z, Horesh D, Ein-Dor T.

Department of Behavioral Sciences, Ariel University Center of Samaria, 40700, Ariel, Israel. gadizy@gmail.com

Abstract

BACKGROUND: The bi-directional relationships between combat-induced posttraumatic symptoms and family relations are yet to be understood. The present study assesses the longitudinal interrelationship of posttraumatic intrusion and avoidance and family cohesion among 208 Israeli combat veterans from the 1982 Lebanon War.

METHODS: Two groups of veterans were assessed with self-report questionnaires 1, 3 and 20 years after the war: a combat stress reaction (CSR) group and a matched non-CSR control group.

RESULTS: Latent Trajectories Modeling showed that veterans of the CSR group reported higher intrusion and avoidance than non-CSR veterans at all three points of time. With time, there was a decline in these symptoms in both groups, but the decline was more salient among the CSR group. The latter also reported lower levels of family cohesion. Furthermore, an incline in family cohesion levels was found in both groups over the years. Most importantly, Autoregressive Cross-Lagged Modeling among CSR and non-CSR veterans revealed that CSR veterans' posttraumatic symptoms in 1983 predicted lower family cohesion in 1985, and lower family cohesion, in turn, predicted posttraumatic symptoms in 2002.

CONCLUSIONS: The findings suggest that psychological breakdown on the battlefield is a marker for future family cohesion difficulties. Our results lend further support to the bi-directional mutual effects of posttraumatic symptoms and family cohesion over time.

PMID: 22752110 [PubMed - in process]

⊕ LinkOut - more resources

12.4.1.2 Analytical Studies

Analytical studies feature non-experimental (observational) questions comparing observations. For example, 'Are women on hormone replacement therapy (HRT) prone to cardiovascular disease than those who are not on HRT?'

1. **Ecological Studies:** Data is assimilated from the existing databases on a particular disease condition and its associated risk factors.

2. **Case-control Studies:** In this study, the clinical scenario is important to draw a relationship between subjects with the disease and without the disease. People with the condition are called cases and they are compared with those without the disease (controls). Figure 12.4 provides the study design for case-control studies.

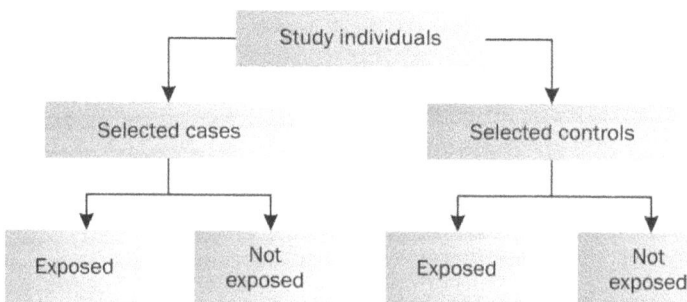

Figure 12.4: Study design for case-control studies.

≳ NCBI   Resources ⊡ How To ⊡

Pub**Med**.gov   PubMed   ⬛
US National Library of Medicine
National Institutes of Health   Advanced

Display Settings: ⊡ Abstract   Send to: ⊡

J Invest Dermatol 2013 Jan 23 doi 10 1036/jid 2013.33 [Epub ahead of print]

Photosensitizing Agents and the Risk of Non-Melanoma Skin Cancer: A Population-Based Case-Control Study.

Robinson SN, Zens MS, Perry AE, Spencer SK, Duell EJ, Karagas MR

Section of Biostatistics and Epidemiology, Department of Community and Family Medicine, The Geisel School of Medicine at Dartmouth, Lebanon, New Hampshire, USA.

Abstract

It is well-known that ultraviolet (UV) light exposure and a sun sensitive phenotype are risk factors for the development of non-melanoma skin cancer (NMSC), including basal cell carcinoma (BCC) and squamous cell carcinoma (SCC). In this New Hampshire population-based case-control study, we collected data from 5,072 individuals, including histologically-confirmed cases of BCC and SCC, and controls via a personal interview to investigate possible associations between photosensitizing medication use and NMSC. After adjustment for potentially confounding factors (e.g. lifetime number of painful sunburns), we found a modest increase in risk of SCC (OR=1.2, 95% CI=1.0-1.4) and BCC (OR=1.2, 95% CI=0.9-1.5), in particular early-onset BCC (≤ 50 years of age) (OR=1.5, 95% CI=1.1-2.1) associated with photosensitizing medication use. For SCC the association was strongest amongst those with tendency to sunburn rather than tan. We also specifically found associations with BCC, and especially early-onset BCC, and photosensitizing antimicrobials. In conclusion, certain commonly prescribed photosensitizing medications may enhance the risk of developing SCC especially in individuals with a sun sensitive phenotype, and may increase the risk of developing BCC and incidence of BCC at a younger age Journal of Investigative Dermatology accepted article preview online, 23 January 2013, doi 10.1038/jid 2013.33

PMC: 23344461 [PubMed - as supplied by publisher]

⊕ LinkOut - more resources

3. **Cross-Sectional, Two Group Studies:** The objective here is to confirm the correlation between the cause and effect. Subjects with and without the effects are observed for the cause, and the possibility of being exposed to the same risk factor is elucidated.

4. **Cohort studies:** In a cohort study, patients are sampled on the basis of exposure and are followed over time, and the occurrence of outcomes is assessed. A cohort study may include a comparison group, although this is not a necessary feature. Cohort study can be prospective or retrospective. Cohort study design is described in Figure 12.5.

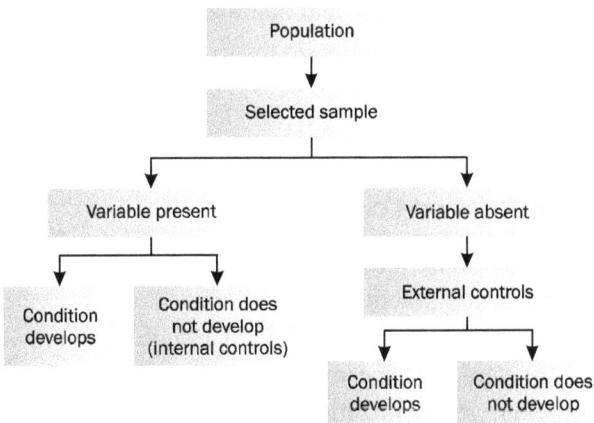

Figure 12.5: Study design for cohort studies.

NCBI   Resources ⊙   How To ⊙

PubMed.gov   PubMed ▾
US National Library of Medicine
National Institutes of Health   Advanced

Display Settings: ⊙ Abstract   Send to: ⊙

Emerg Med J. 2013 Jan 23. [Epub ahead of print]
Emergency medical admissions, deaths at weekends and the public holiday effect. Cohort study.
Smith S, Allan A, Greenlaw N, Finlay S, Isles C
Medical Unit, Dumfries and Galloway Royal Infirmary, Dumfries, UK.

Abstract
OBJECTIVES: To assess whether mortality of patients admitted on weekends and public holidays was higher in a district general hospital whose consultants are present more than 6 h per day on the acute medical unit with no other fixed clinical commitments.
DESIGN: Cohort study.
SETTING: Secondary care.
PARTICIPANTS: All emergency medical admissions to Dumfries and Galloway Royal Infirmary between 1 January 2008 and 31 December 2010.
METHODS: We examined 7 and 30 day mortality for all weekend and for all public holiday admissions, using all weekday and non-public holiday admissions, respectively, as comparators. We adjusted mortality for age, gender, comorbidity, deprivation, diagnosis and year of admission.
RESULTS: 771 (3.8%) of 20,072 emergency admissions died within 7 days of admission and 1780 (8.9%) within 30 days. Adjusted weekend mortality in the all weekend versus all other days analysis was not significantly higher at 7 days (OR 1.10, 95% CI 0.92 to 1.31; p=0.312) or at 30 days (OR 1.07, 95% CI 0.94 to 1.21; p=0.322). By contrast, adjusted public holiday mortality in the all public holidays versus all other days analysis was 48% higher at 7 days (OR 1.48, 95% CI 1.12 to 1.95; p=0.006) and 27% higher at 30 days (OR 1.27, 95% CI 1.02 to 1.57; p=0.031). Interactions between the weekend variable and the public holiday variable were not statistically significant for mortality at either 7 or 30 days.
CONCLUSIONS: Patients admitted as emergencies to medicine on public holidays had significantly higher mortality at 7 and 30 days compared with patients admitted on other days of the week.

PMID: 23345314 [PubMed - as supplied by publisher]

⊕ LinkOut - more resources

12.4.2 Experimental/Interventional Studies

These studies are called trials because they provide results on experimentation with an intervention on subjects. Trial designs are classified on the basis of the pattern of treatment/intervention allocation.

1. Randomized vs. Non-randomized studies

2. Matched-pair analysis and cross-over trials

3. Single blind, double blind, and open-label randomized studies

4. Prospective vs. retrospective studies

5. Phase I, II, III, IV studies

6. Postmarketing survey

12.4.2.1   Randomized Control Trials

Randomized control trials (RCTs) generate gold standard evidence for evidence-based clinical practice. In randomized studies, the treatment allocation is done randomly (Figure 12.6). Through randomization, all the subjects have the same chance of being assigned to each of the study groups. Additionally, randomization ensures comparability between the study groups in terms of known/unknown factors and measurable/

unmeasurable factors. Randomized control trial is the only design that can prove efficacy, benefits/risks of a particular treatment/intervention. RCTs significantly influence clinical practice. RCTs are mandatory for obtaining FDA approval for new drugs or devices. Randomization eliminates bias in allocating treatment and ensures the validity of the statistical significance of tests. There are different types of randomization: simple, blocked, stratified, adaptive, and cluster.

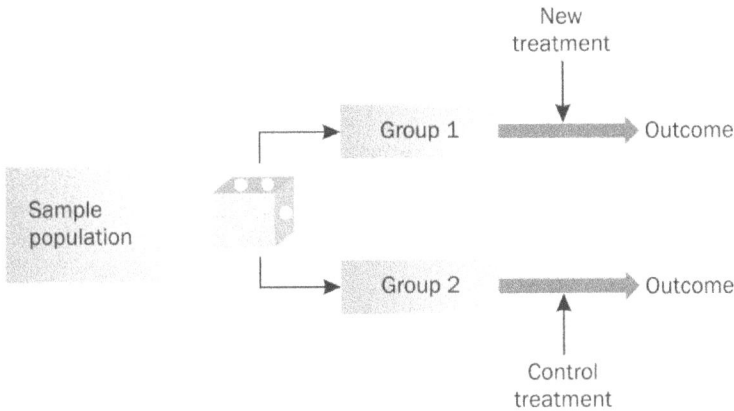

Figure 12.6: Randomized control trial design.

12.4.2.2 Matched-pair Analysis and Cross-over Study

When randomization is not possible, two methods can be used to minimize the effect of extraneous variables: matched-pair analysis and the cross-over method. In a matched-pair analysis, subjects in both the experimental and control groups are 'paired' on the factor or factors of interest, e.g., age-matched controls (Figure 12.7). In the cross-over method, the subjects, upon completion of one treatment, are switched to another (or none) (Figure 12.8). In this manner, the subjects serve as their 'own controls.'

12.4.2.3 Single-blind, Double-blind, and Open-label Randomized Studies

In order to minimize researcher bias, clinical trials are often 'blinded.' In the single-blind method, either the observer(s) or the patient(s) is kept ignorant of the group to which the subjects are assigned. In the double-blind method both the subjects and investigators are unaware of who is actually getting which specific treatment. Open label study is the opposite of the double-blind study. In this method, patients and investigators both know the intervention they are receiving.

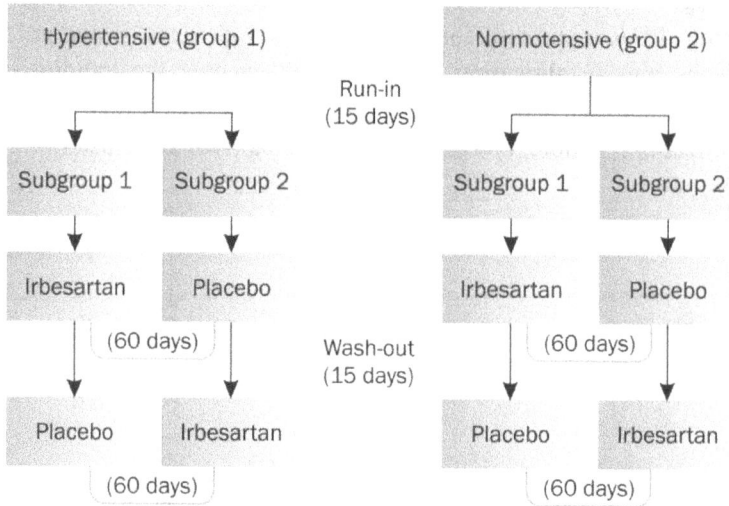

Figure 12.7: Matched- pair study design.

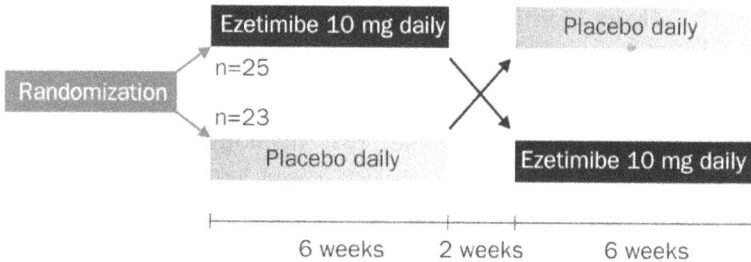

Figure 12.8: Cross-over study.

12.4.2.4   Prospective vs. Retrospective Studies

In a prospective design, the researcher follows participants and measures or observes for future events or end points. In a retrospective design, the researcher analyzes data after the event/end point for a disease and classifies the participants simultaneously into the group categories. If there are only two categories such as yes (case) and no (control) groups, it is called a case-control study. If there are more than two categories, it is called a cross-sectional study.

12.4.3 Phase I, II, III, IV Trials

The FDA model for approval of new drugs, devices, or procedures defines four phases of clinical trials, each with a different purpose:

- **Phase I Clinical Trials** involve studies performed to evaluate the safety of diagnostic, therapeutic, or prophylactic drugs, devices, or techniques in healthy subjects and to determine the safe dosage range (if appropriate). These tests also are used to determine pharmacologic and pharmacokinetic properties (toxicity, metabolism, absorption, elimination, and preferred route of administration). They involve a small number of persons and usually last for about 1 year.

- **Phase II Clinical Trials** involve studies that are usually controlled to assess the effectiveness and dosage (if appropriate) of diagnostic, therapeutic, or prophylactic drugs, devices, or techniques. These studies are performed on several hundred volunteers, including a limited number of patients with the target disease or disorder, and last about two years.

- **Phase III Clinical Trials** are comparative studies designed to verify the effectiveness of diagnostic, therapeutic, or prophylactic drugs, devices, or techniques determined in phase II studies. During these trials, patients are monitored closely by physicians to identify any adverse reactions from long-term use. These studies are performed on groups of patients large enough to identify clinically significant responses and usually last about three years.

- **Phase IV Clinical Trials** are planned post-marketing studies of diagnostic, therapeutic, or prophylactic drugs, devices, or techniques that have been approved for general sale. These studies are often conducted to obtain additional data about the safety and efficacy of a product.

Chapter - 13

Get an Overview of the Subject even before Understanding the Topic

Before you begin to understand the topic that you are assigned to write, you should have an overview of the subject/specialty or disease you are writing on. For example, if you are writing on metformin, you should know everything about diabetes, like its epidemiology, causes, complications, treatment options available, advantages and disadvantages of each class and individual molecule used for diabetes treatment. A review article (for example from the journal, DRUGS of ADIS publication, Expert opinion, or American Family Physician) related to the subject is sufficient to get an overview of the topic. Only then, would it be possible for you to write an article on metformin.

Do not read articles only for the purpose of getting information alone. Observe each article for the style of writing, how a writer discusses a topic, headings and subheadings, logical flow of the article, and tables and figures. In addition, read non-medical books, journals, and newsletter for better understanding of the style of writing, grammar, style of presentation, etc.

Most of the reading can happen while resourcing itself. Once you have understood the topic, next step is to write an outline.

Chapter - 14

Content Approach or Outline

O nce you understand the topic and references, next step is to write an outline. Outline is like a skeleton of the body. It is like a map of the city for a traveller. Outline gives structured approach and logical flow to the article. Outline also reflects your understanding of the topic assigned to you and the references that you have collected. Outline differs for different types of articles. For original research articles, outline typically comprises of IMRAD (Introduction, Method, Result and Discussion). For case reports, it is case presentation, and discussion. However, for review articles and medical communication articles, there is no fixed format. You may think that drafting an outline takes a lot of time and you can write the article as well in the same time. In fact, preparing an outline first saves time than writing without one. Main purposes of outline are:

- To assist you in the process of writing
- To help you organize your ideas
- To present your material in a logical form
- To correlate the ideas in your writing
- To construct an ordered overview of your writing
- To define boundaries and groups

Some writers call the outline as 'content approach' or table of contents (TOC). I think using the term TOC for outline is inappropriate. Outline is what you want to write; it is drafted in the beginning. TOC is what you have written; it is written at the end. A glance through the content outline is sufficient for the readers to decide to read or chuck it! The outline is the door/window to your article.

The headings and subheadings of content outline should be:

- Descriptive of the subject that you are going to discuss

- Together, the headings and subheadings should provide a structure to the article that you are going to write
- Drive the core message

Usually, headings and subheadings given in content approach are self-explanatory. If required, write one or two sentences for each heading and subheading on what you want to write. That will give a better idea for building the content while writing or discussing with the client for getting the approval. Once the outline is ready, next step is to start actual writing. As you proceed to write within the scope of the outline, the article takes a shape.

Content Approach

Example 1: Role of tranexamic acid in gastrointestinal bleeding

- Incidence of upper GI bleeding
- Consequences
- Treatment options
- Efficacy of tranexamic acid
  - ➢ Reduction in bleeding at endoscopy
  - ➢ Reduction in rebleeding
  - ➢ Reduction in need for surgery
  - ➢ Reduction in mortality
- Safety
- Guideline recommendations
- Summary
- References

Content Approach

Example 2: An overview of the guidelines on male sexual dysfunction: Premature ejaculation.

- Introduction
- Epidemiology
- Influence of premature ejaculation on Quality of life (QoL)
- Risk factors
- Classification
  - ➢ New classification—premature ejaculation syndromes

- Diagnosis
  - ➢ Medical and sexual history
  - ➢ Premature ejaculation assessment questionnaires
    - ✓ Premature ejaculation diagnostic tool (PEDT)
    - ✓ Arabic Index of premature ejaculation (AIPE)
    - ✓ Premature ejaculation profile (PEP)
    - ✓ Intravaginal ejaculatory latency time (IELT)
  - ➢ Physical examination and other tests
- Management of premature ejaculation
  - ➢ Psychological/behavioral strategies
  - ➢ Topical anesthetic agents
  - ➢ Pharmacological therapy
    - ✓ Implication of central dopaminergic neurotransmission in ejaculation: An overview
      - Selective serotonin reuptake inhibitors
      - Dapoxetine
      - Phosphodiesterase type 5 inhibitors
      - Other drugs
- Summary
- References

Chapter - 15

Writing Different Parts of the Article

Initially, we had a problem in including this section in the book. The dilemma was should we share our ideas on what we perceive in writing these sections or look into standard good books and write it like an article. After much debate, we decided to write what we learnt and practice to do. As this book is conceived based on our experience and experiments, we decided to share our views on how we typically write. Any article will follow a logical flow. Unlike an original research paper that follows the IMRD (introduction, Method, Results and Discussion) style, a customized medical article encompasses:

- Title
- Introduction
- Body of content
- Highlighting points
- Summary/conclusion
- References

There are no hard and fast rules for writing each of the sections of the article. It varies from article to article, subject to subject and writer to writer. For better understanding of the topic, do not hesitate to discuss with your team lead or a co-medical writer as to how you are planning to write the article.

> *We usually draw an analogy between an article and a movie. Similar to the dramatic introduction of the hero/heroine in a movie, introduction should be interesting. Like a good script interlinking the characters, write the body of content without any hitch. Figures and tables are like the songs in the movies, they add value to the article. The highlighting points are like comedians. Like a good ending of a movie, an article should have good summary or conclusion.*

15.1   Writing an Introduction

Introduction is a revelation to the remaining section of the article that you are writing. The style of writing introduction is dependent on the individual medical writers' perception of the topic. Nevertheless, the content written in introduction should draw the attention of the reader (interesting), provide clarity, and be informative and logical without any ambiguity. As far as possible quote, the latest references in the introduction.

Ideally, an introduction should

- Announce the topic
- Limit to the topic
- Indicate a plan
- Catch the reader's attention
- Establish tone and point of view

The length of the introduction depends on the length of the article. For a booklet of 8-12 pages, introduction can be up to 1 page. For articles for newsletter or brochures (4 pages) one paragraph (8-10 lines) introduction is sufficient. A typical introduction written by me (if the article is focusing on a drug for a particular condition) would be covering the following aspects:

- Incidence or prevalence of disease
- Mortality and morbidity of the disease
- Available treatment options
- Disadvantages with the available options or treatment gaps and need for another drug.
- Availability of new drug or new class of drug
- How the new drug is useful in overcoming treatment gap or disadvantages of other options.

It is also better to write one or two sentence about the points that are going to be covered in the article. You can add variety to introduction by beginning the introduction in different ways:

- A quotation (ensure that its relevance is explained or self-explanatory)

- A question
- An acknowledgment of an opinion opposite to the one you plan to take
- A very short narrative or anecdote that has a direct bearing on your paper
- An interesting fact
- A definition or explanation of a term relevant to your paper
- Irony or paradox
- An analogy (ensure it is original but not too far-fetched)

15.2 Writing the Body of the Article

Body of an article is not stereotypical; it is very subjective and is dependent on the understanding and writing skill of a writer. The body of the article comprises:

- Headings and subheadings
- Paragraphs relevant to headings and subheadings
- Tables and illustrations (figures)
- Highlighting points

Revise the headings and subheadings created at the time of framing the content outline while writing the body of the article, if required. The body of an article will be an elaborate of the content outline. The style of writing and the references used should be relevant at any given point. A better understanding of each section of the outline will help you to write a good content. Each line should be interconnected and paragraphs should be meaningful. There should be appropriate link/transition between paragraphs and headings and subheadings. Do not alter the meaning of the original article statements while paraphrasing the information. Support the content with figures and tables. Be consistent in using acronyms and abbreviations and elaborate them in their first occurrence. There are style guides, which can be used as a reference to ensure consistency in the article.

The body of the article:

- Should have paragraphs that are meaningful, relevant and written effectively
- There should be a smooth transition/link between paragraphs or headings/subheadings
- Data should be displayed as graphs/tables/algorithms/illustrations, wherever possible
- Should follow a proper style guide for consistency

15.2.1   Art of Writing

A paragraph is the basic unit of any article. A paragraph is a group of sentences related to ONE topic. Its main function is to present meaningful information related to one topic that is easy to read. Each sentence within the paragraph should not lengthy. The idea a writer wants to convey in a paragraph can be expressed in one sentence. That sentence is called topic sentence. It is the most important part of a paragraph. Correlate the sentences within a paragraph to reflect the topic sentence. Structure of a paragraph is similar to a big article. It should have an introduction (topic sentence), main body and a conclusion. Paragraph should have coherence and flow. Coherence means that ideas fit together. Flow means that interlinked sentences without any gaps in the idea discussed. A paragraph will be coherent when all the sentences correlate to one topic. Relevance alone is not sufficient to establish coherence. You have to arrange all the sentences related to topic in a logical order/sequence to get flow. Flow can be achieved by 2 methods:

- Suppose you are going to discuss 2-3 topics at the beginning of the paragraph. E.g., There are 3 risk factors; first and major risk factor is age, second is smoking and third is diet. In this example, first sentence not only talks about the topic, it introduces each factor with terms like first, second, etc., you can use digits instead of words.
- Interlink the sentences. It is not possible to number the parts of paragraph in all the cases. In such cases, maintain the flow by connecting the sentences within a paragraph.

Length of the paragraph depends on the topic, nature of writing and the reader. Lengthy paragraphs make the reader 'fatigue'. Very short paragraphs imply that the topic is not well elaborated. A paragraph should have minimum three sentences. Think about forming a new paragraph if you have written 6-7 sentences.

15.2.2   Framing Tables

Tables are list of words and numbers. They are useful to represent complex data in an easy to read format. Tables reduce number of sentences in the text. Moreover, they add value to the article presentation. Tables should not duplicate the content written in the text. Typical components of a table is depicted in Table 15.1. You can create tables in any of the following ways.

Table 15.1 Parts of the table

- Tables can be created from the available data in the original reference
- Tables can be adopted from the original reference with some modifications to avoid copyright issues.
- Sometimes, the data given in two or more figures can be converted into table (when space is a constraint for including all the figures).

Pay attention to the following details while creating tables from the data

- Tables should be self-explanatory
- Write appropriate table captions
- The table content should be grouped appropriately
- Mention the units of measurement along with the parameters
- If the table contains data from various references, then quote the references in the table footnote or in the text where the table is cited
- Give all acronyms and abbreviations used in the tables as a footnote within the table
- Cite the table in the right place in the text
- Cite the references for the table in the text where the table is cited
- Insert references in a separate column, if required; however, it increases number of columns and occupies more space. Alternatively you can give references in the footnote of the table

15.2.3   Creating Illustrations

Illustrations or figures are visual representation of data. Figures give breathing space and attractive look to the designed article. They simplify the context of content. Moreover, the ease of converting data into graphs and algorithms shows the confidence and understanding of the subject by the medical writer. Clients appreciate simplification of data through figures. Therefore, you should intersperse articles with figures. Always remember to give appropriate figure captions. The captions should be able to communicate the content independently. There are various kinds of figures (but all of them are referred to as figures in the article).

15.2.4   Illustrations

Illustrations are useful to show anatomy and to explain physiology or microscopic changes. They are also useful to show mechanism of action (Figure 15.1).

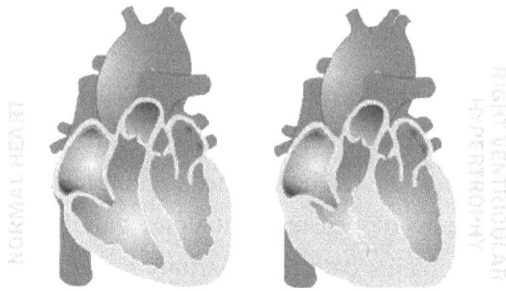

Figure 15.1: Illustration showing a healthy heart (left) and right ventricular hypertrophy (right).

15.2.5 Photos

Photos are usually depicted in case reports (Figure 15.2).

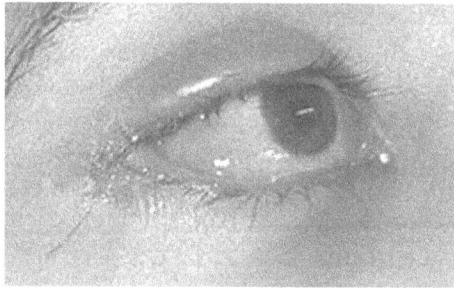

Figure 15.2: Photograph of a patient with allergic conjunctivitis.

15.2.6 Flow Charts (Algorithms)

Algorithms are useful to show decision tree and classification (Figures 15.3 and 15.4).

15.2.7 Graphs

Graphs are graphical representation of data. The type of charts differ based the data.

- Line graph (Figure 15.5)
- Bar graph (Figure 15.6)
- Pie chart (Figure 15.7)
- Kaplan Meyer graph (Figure 15.8)

- Forest plot (Figure 15.9)
- L'Abbé plot (Figure 15.10)

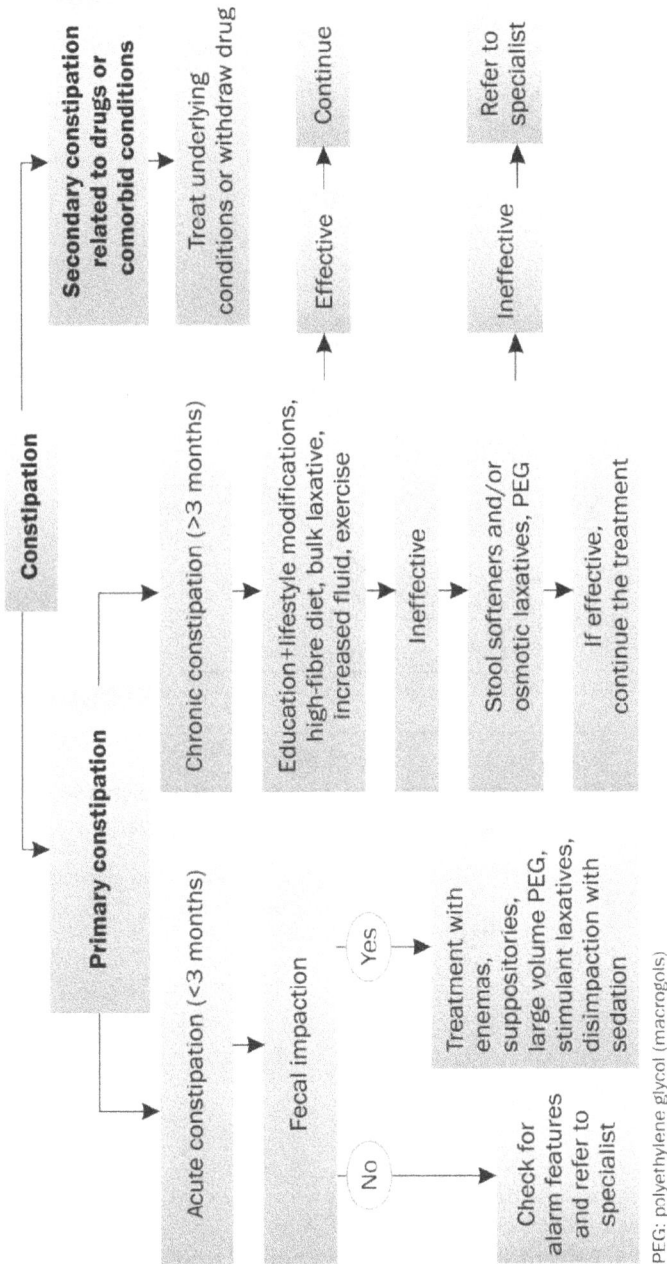

Figure 15.3: Treatment algorithm for constipation.

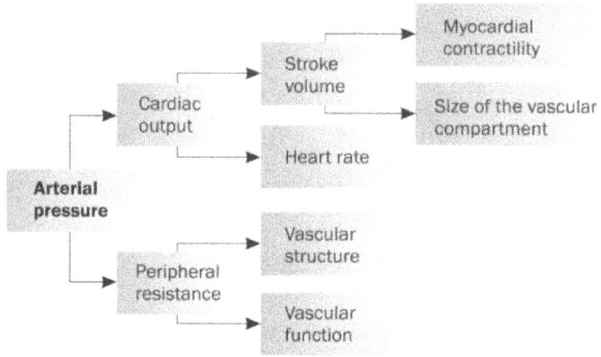

Figure 15.4: Flowchart explaining factors affecting arterial pressure.

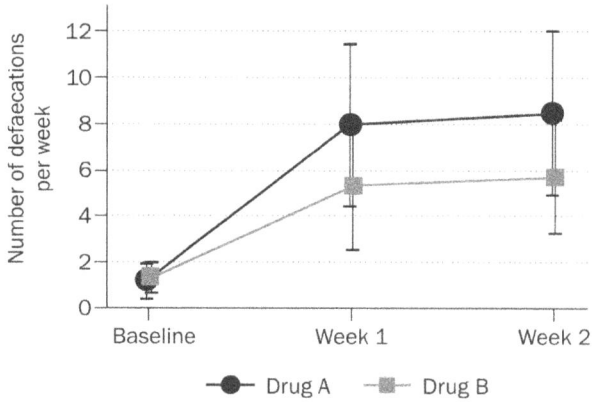

Figure 15.5: Defecation frequency drug A plus electrolytes was higher than drug B in patients with chronic constipation.

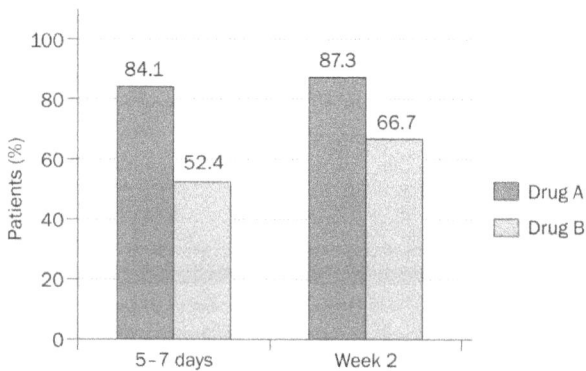

Figure 15.6: Percentage of patients with normal stool form, following treatment with drug A was significantly higher vs. drug B.

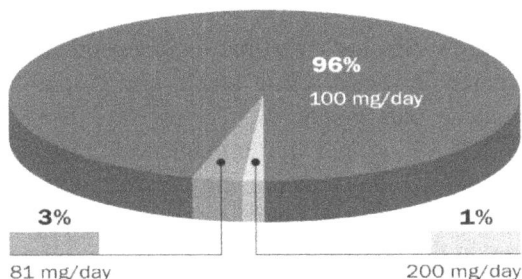

Figure 15.7: Dose of aspirin consumed by the patients in a study.

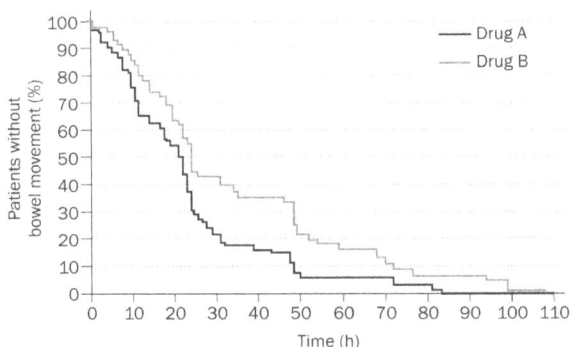

Figure 15.8: Time to first bowel movement following treatment with low-dose drug A plus electrolytes twice-daily or drug B twice-daily in patients with chronic constipation.

Review: Drug A verses drug B for chronic constipation

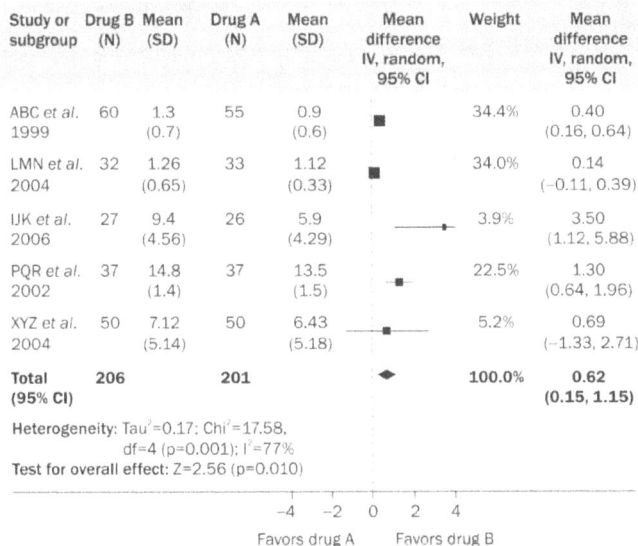

Study or subgroup	Drug B (N)	Mean (SD)	Drug A (N)	Mean (SD)	Mean difference IV, random, 95% CI	Weight	Mean difference IV, random, 95% CI
ABC et al. 1999	60	1.3 (0.7)	55	0.9 (0.6)	■	34.4%	0.40 (0.16, 0.64)
LMN et al. 2004	32	1.26 (0.65)	33	1.12 (0.33)	■	34.0%	0.14 (-0.11, 0.39)
IJK et al. 2006	27	9.4 (4.56)	26	5.9 (4.29)		3.9%	3.50 (1.12, 5.88)
PQR et al. 2002	37	14.8 (1.4)	37	13.5 (1.5)		22.5%	1.30 (0.64, 1.96)
XYZ et al. 2004	50	7.12 (5.14)	50	6.43 (5.18)		5.2%	0.69 (-1.33, 2.71)
Total (95% CI)	206		201		◆	100.0%	0.62 (0.15, 1.15)

Heterogeneity: Tau^2=0.17; Chi^2=17.58, df=4 (p=0.001); I^2=77%
Test for overall effect: Z=2.56 (p=0.010)

-4   -2   0   2   4
Favors drug A   Favors drug B

Figure 15.9: Forest plot of stool frequency per week for drug A and drug B.

Line graphs are useful to show changes overtime. If independent and dependent variables are numeric, then use a line graph. Bar graphs are useful to compare two or more parameters. Bar graphs are used to represent discrete, grouped data of ordinal or nominal scale. Use pie charts to show proportion. Graphs can be created using the chart option in MS Word or Excel sheet. It is better to create chart in the word because it gives the scope for editors to edit the data, if required.

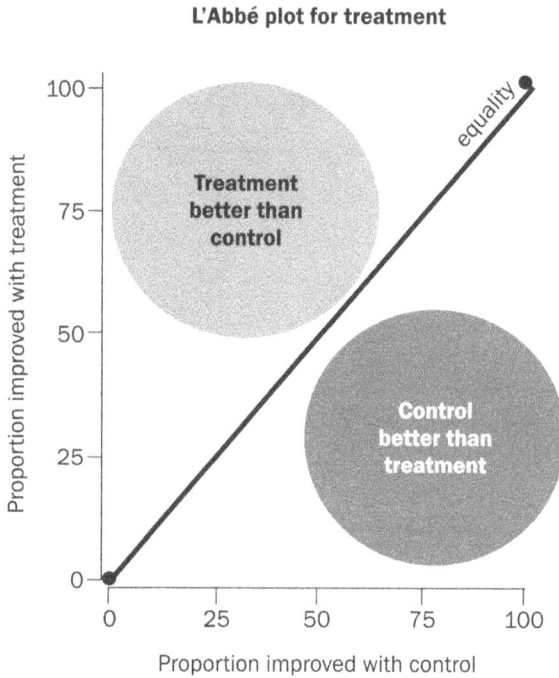

Figure 15.10: L'Abbé plot showing proportion of patients responding to treatment or placebo.

Every table and figure should have a caption that describes the content in easy manner and is standalone. You can write figure/table captions in different ways.

15.3 Writing Summary and Conclusion

Summary and conclusion are different. Summary is short version of the article and has important points of the article. On the other hand, conclusion has key points of research findings in a research article. Conclusion gives the scope for writing the opinion of the writer. Reading a summary should give you the gist of the article. Write summary in a paragraph or in bullet points. Do not discuss or write ideas that are not covered in the whole of the article in the summary. Citing references for summary or conclusion is not required. However, some clients would ask to cite references for summary and conclusion too! In general, giving a reference in conclusion means that you are not sure and that you are writing someone else's conclusion.

15.4 Write Catchy/Interesting Titles

Why do we discuss writing title in end? In fact, you can write better title for the article at the end of writing than at the beginning. Write a tentative title while beginning and modify or change the title after completing. Readers spend maximum 2 seconds looking at the title and decide whether to read your article or not. Therefore, title should be impressive at the first look. Title should give an indication about the topic of the article and elicit interest. It should be complete and eye catching. Take clues from the articles that you read for understanding or as references.

15.5 References and Reference Citation

Medical writers are not fiction writers. Every point written in the article should have a supporting reference. Other purposes of citing reference are

- Evidence-based or authenticity to the content
- If any reader wants more information, they can refer the original article
- To give credit to the original author

A reference is the address of an article; it is unique. There are two components in writing references.

- **In-text citation:** The reference numbers are given in the content against the supporting data
- **Listing of references:** The reference is given at the end of the article that corresponds to the citation in the text.

15.5.1 In-text Citation

There are different styles for in-text citation and listing references. However, the purpose of referencing is to provide the readers the details of published article in a particular journal/book/conference for their further study.

- In the Modern Language Association (MLA) style, the in-text citation carries Author's name followed by a space and the relevant page number(s).

  Eg. Human beings have been described as "symbol-using animals" (Burke 3)

- While in the American Psychological Association (APA) style, the in-text citation carries the Author's name followed by a space and the year of publishing.

  Eg. Human beings have been described as "symbol-using animals" (Burke 1998)

- Vancouver and American Medical Association (AMA) style are same, except that in the Vancouver style, the in-text citation is given within parenthesis, while in the AMA, the references are given as superscripts

Vancouver style

Eg., Human beings have been described as "symbol-using animals". [4]

AMA style

E.g., Human beings have been described as "symbol-using animals".[4]

Different disciplines follow different style for referencing (Table 15.2). In general, for all medicomarketing writing, we use the Vancouver style with slight modification.

Table 15.2: Referencing style for different disciplines

Reference style	Discipline
APA	Psychology, education, and other social sciences
MLA	Literature, arts, and humanities
AMA/Vancouver	Medicine, health, and biological sciences
Turabian	Designed for college students to use with all subjects
Chicago	Used with all subjects in the 'real world' by books, magazines, newspapers, and other non-scholarly publications

MLA, Modern Language Association; APA, American Psychological Association; AMA, American Medical Association

15.5.2 Listing of References

In MLA style and APA style, references are listed in alphabetical order. In Vancouver and AMA style, all references cited in the text are listed in numerical order. In the list, you need to write about the source of article. In general, following information about the reference is required to write the cited article.

- Who is the author?
- What is the title of the article?
- In which journal or publication was it published?
- When was it published?
- What is the volume number
- What are the printed pages?

15.5.3 Examples for Writing References According to AMA/Vancouver Style

15.5.3.1 Books

Single author: Shepard TH. Catalog of Teratogenic Agents. 7th ed. Baltimore, Md: Johns Hopkins Press; 1992.

More than one author: List all authors if six or less, otherwise list first three followed by 'et al.' Baselt RC, Cravey RH. Disposition of Toxic Drugs and Chemicals in Man. 4th ed. Foster City, Calif: Chemical Toxicology Institute; 1995.

Book–with editors: Armitage JO, Antman KH, eds. High-dose Cancer Therapy: Pharmacology, Hematopoietins, Stem Cells. Baltimore, Md: Williams & Wilkins; 1995.

Chapter from a book: Degner LF, McWilliams ME. Challenges in conducting cross-national nursing research. In: Fitzpatrick JJ, Stevenson JS, Polis NS, eds. Nursing Research and its Utilization: International State of the Science. New York, NY: Springer; 1994:211–215.

15.5.3.2 Journals

Single author: Moldofsky H. Sleep, neuroimmune and neuroendocrine functions in fibromyalgia and chronic fatigue syndrome. Adv Neuroimmunol. 1995;5:39-56.

More than one author: List all authors if six or less, otherwise list first three followed by "et al." Raux H, Coulon P, Lafay F, Flamand A. Monoclonal antibodies which recognizes the acidic configuration of the rabies glycoprotein at the surface of the virion can be neutralizing. Virology. 1995; 210:400–408.

Monographic series: Davidoff RA. Migraine: Manifestations, Pathogenesis, and Management. Philadelphia, Pa: FA Davis; 1995. Contemporary Neurology Series, No. 42.

Online journals with volume and page information: Simon JA, Hudes ES. Relationship of ascorbic acid to blood lead levels. JAMA [serial online]. 1999; 281:2289-2293. Available from: http://jama.ama-assn.org/content/281/24/2289. full.pdf+html. Accessed on October 31, 2011.

Online journals without volume and page information: Gordon GF. Bypassing heart surgery. Alternative Medicine [serial online]. July 1999; issue 30.

15.5.3.3 Paper Presented at a Meeting

Colon HM, Robles RR, Marrero CA, et al. Frequency of drug injection in Puerto Rico and among Puerto Rican injection drug users compared to other ethnic groups and geographical regions. Paper presented at: American Public Health Association Annual Meeting; October 30-November 3, 1994; Washington, DC.

15.5.3.4 Online Website

Terre Haute Center for Medical Education. The THCME Medical Biochemistry page. Available at: http://web.indstate.edu/ thcme/mwking/ home.html. Accessed August 24, 1999.

15.5.3.5 When to Cite References

Do not reference each line of the text, but at the most, each of the paragraphs should bear one reference citation. Importantly, cite references when you are providing

- statistical or epidemiological data;
- authors name
- guidelines
- definitions
- figures/tables/algorithms

Chapter - 16

Revision

Most of us cannot write perfectly or I would say near-perfectly in the first attempt. Drafting is a spontaneous and active. You cannot simultaneously concentrate on flow of the article and grammar, spelling, punctuation and figure/table citations. Therefore, draft requires revision/rewriting. Revision involves correcting grammatical and spelling mistakes and rewriting wherever necessary. Always revise your document one day after the first draft. A break in between writing and revision gives you ample time to clear the topic from your thoughts and so the next time you read, you will be able to identify the gap or missing link or flaw in flow of the article. With respect to grammar, you will read the article with 'minds eye' than actually reading, if you revise immediately after writing the first draft.

16.1 Points to be Taken Care While Reviewing the Article

Ask the following questions while reviewing the article.

- Is it according to the brief?
- What is the client's product?
- Who are the target audience?
- USP of brand/generic
- Is it conveying the message client wants?
- Is the article lengthy? Or short? Number of characters or pages?
- Is the title interesting?
- Is the introduction introducing the topic?
- Are you giving clues to what you are going to discuss in the article?
- Are the sentences short?

- Is there link between the sentences?
- Is paragraph intact?
- Can we convert some data into table or figure?
- Are the paragraph lengthy?
- Is the article fluid/progressing/transition/story?
- Are there any contradictory statements at different places?
- Are there any ambiguous/unclear/confusing/vague sentences?
- Are the heading and subheadings interesting?
- Is the text under heading and subheading relevant?
- Are important studies/references used?
- Are figures/tables quoted at right place?
- Are figures and tables relevant to text?
- Is the figure/table caption interesting/different from original?
- Are there any repetition of text?
- Are highlighting points appropriate?
- Is the conclusion reflecting the article?

If 'yes' the answer for all these questions, then the article would meet the requirement.

PART - III

Variety of Medicomarketing Projects

Pharmaceutical companies constantly require scientific inputs for marketing their brand. The variety of medicomarketing projects include:

- *Teaser campaign*
- *Training kit (Slides and Manual)*
- *Product monograph*
- *Detail aid or visual aid*
- *Symposium highlights*
- *Advisory board meetings*
- *Brochures*
- *Newsletters*
- *Pharmaceutical brand website*
- *Content for media*
- *Patient education materials*

Chapter - 17

Teaser Campaign

Before launching a product in to the market, the advertisements build the need, curiosity, interest and/or excitement about the new product. Such advertisements are called teaser campaigns. They tease the public by offering only small amount of information without revealing either the sponsor of the advertisement or the product being advertised. This strategy is applicable for pharmaceutical brands also.

17.1 Writing for Teaser Campaign

Teaser campaigns are usually taken care by the advertising agencies. It involves lot of creativity. The idea may be simple but has to be packaged in an interesting, appealing and relevant manner.

> **Example 1:** A company wanting to launch telmisartan focused morning blood pressure surge (MBPS) control by telmisartan as its unique selling potential (USP). They created a series of brochures and advertisements highlighting the need to control MBPS, without mentioning the generic name or brand before the launch to create awareness about MBPS. A series of topics proposed for the teaser campaign include:

- There is an increased risk for heart attack, stroke, and sudden death in the first few hours of the morning

- Cardiovascular events occur most frequently in the morning

- Most commonly used antihypertensives are not able to control BP in the morning

- Antihypertensive agents taken once daily in the morning, the timing of the trough plasma drug level, and thereby the lowest pharmacodynamic effect, often coincides with the early morning rise in blood pressure and heart rate

Morning BP Predicts Stroke

Montreal: Hypertension in the morning hours is a strong, independent predictor of future stroke events in elderly patients say researchers. The morning blood pressure (BP) has greater risk than even sustained hypertension. Another study from the same researchers claims that a morning surge in blood pressure is a better predictor of stroke than extreme dips in pressure during the night. Stroke risk in the "extreme dippers" was highest only when this characteristic was combined with a morning surge in blood pressure. These reports were presented by XYZ, MD, at the HHH Scientific Sessions 2002.

Example 2: When Pfizer wanted to launch tranexamic acid (cyclokapron) injection, they first highlighted the hazards of bleeding during surgery and blood transfusion, to emphasize the need to control/reduce bleeding during surgery.

Chapter - 18

Training Kit (Slides and Manual)

Training manual might be for the doctors as a part of continuing medical education (CME) or for medical representatives. The PowerPoint slides are delivered in a compact disc or in the form of any of the electronic media. Training manual may be in printed (booklet) or electronic (online or interactive) versions.

Medical representatives: The objective is to train the field force before the launch of a drug. The content has to be as simple as possible.

Doctors: The objective is to update the doctors on the latest developments, in case of existing brands. As a part of product launch strategy, the training kits provide the complete information on the new molecule.

18.1 Writing Training Kit Inputs

Training kits provides an opportunity to reveal the creative side of the writer. There are different ways to approach the presentation. Here, subject knowledge, understanding and creativity go hand in hand. There are two parts: one is the slides in PowerPoint and the other is the print manual supplementing the slides. The print manual is the speaker notes or supplement or the guidebook for the slides.

- First, prepare the PowerPoint slides and then write the content for the manual.
- Like any other kind of writing, create a content approach and then allocate the number of slides for each section. The content approach for a new launch molecule will be more or less similar to the product monograph

- Get the client approval for content approach
- Wherever there is a scope for creating animation (especially mechanism of action) get the animator to design the animation without any mistakes
- Design simple templates according to the brand colors. If design is complex, then the content will be lost in the design background and reader might lose focus
- For consistency and esthetic look, after the client approval, get the tables, figures or algorithms designed uniformly
- Use authentic journals, books and data on file (occasionally) references only
- As with any PowerPoint presentation,
  - ➢ the content in each slide should not be more than four lines
  - ➢ use simple language
  - ➢ it should be pictorial; the graphs and tables should be self-explanatory
- The manual is written once the client approves the slides
- The manual also contains frequently asked questions (FAQs) and prescribing information.

Chapter - 19

Product Monograph

When a product is introduced in to the market, it is essential to give comprehensive information about the product to the doctors. Hence, a 'Product Monograph' describing the pharmacology, indications, clinical efficacy, tolerability etc., is useful to provide information to the doctors.

19.1   Writing a Product Monograph

A product monograph may not highlight any particular USP of the drug. Although information provided in a product monograph is comprehensive, it is not elaborate. Product monograph is not a review article. It contains less text and more figures and tables. Information should be presented in a crisp format. Design and layout should be attractive. Product monograph may be as big as 50-80 pages.

Do not get confused with monographs distributed by the companies with product monographs published in the drug information books and product monographs published for regulatory purpose in Canada. These monographs are different from the monographs in the drug information books and regulatory monographs in the following ways. Product monographs published in the drug information books and product monographs published for regulatory purpose are like prescribing information. They are more technical in terms of content. A typical product monograph for brand promotion as a marketing input for launch contains crisp information and is design oriented.

For a typical table of content of the product monograph given below, you can write the content comprehensively for each section. The amount of content for each section should be decided and allot more number of pages for the clinical pharmacology section.

- Introduction
- Rationale
- Composition of the brand
- Product/drug description - chemistry
- Clinical pharmacology
  - ➢ Pharmacodynamics
  - ➢ Pharmacokinetics
  - ➢ Summary
- Preclinical data
- Clinical Efficacy
  - ➢ Summary of clinical studies
- Indications
- Safety and tolerability
  - ➢ Summary of clinical safety studies
- Dosage and administration
  - ➢ Dosage
  - ➢ Administration
- Conclusions
- References

Introduction: Disease or the drug itself is the topic sentence for this section. Some product monographs begin with positioning of the brand. They may discuss the epidemiology of the disease. For e.g., A product monograph on Curosurf, a porcine-derived surfactant for management of neonatal respiratory distress syndrome, begins with the epidemiology of the problem, and then discusses management, available surfactants, then about Curosurf.

Rationale: Atleast one page should give evidence-based reasons for using/launching the drug or a combination of drug in a particular medical condition. In fact, the unique selling potential (USP) of the molecule can also be considered as the key for writing the rationale. This section is most important as it links the introduction to the subsequent sections.

Composition of the brand: Give information of the drug/drug combination along with the strength.

Product or drug description: Discuss chemistry and chemical structure of the drug in this section.

Clinical pharmacology: In this section, discuss the mechanism of action, the ADME (absorption, distribution, metabolism, and elimination) and drug interactions.

Writing RATIONALE in a Product Monograph

Example 1: Deflazacort was launched in India by Alkem in 2008. Although the molecule was old, Alkem launched deflazacort for the first time in India. As an initial marketing support, a product monograph was developed. Unlike the typical corticosteroids, deflazacort apparently does not affect the hypothalamus-cortical axis. This USP was the rationale in the product monograph.

Example 2: In a product monograph on ceftriazone/tazobactam, the rationale is the use of a beta-lactam and beta-lactamase inhibitor combination to overcome beta-lactamase mediated resistance in microbes. Beta-lactamase inhibitors bind irreversibly to the beta-lactamases, render them inactive, and hence spare the beta-lactam antibiotic.

Preclinical data: This section is optional and is usually not included in the product monograph, unless there is a specific need.

Clinical efficacy: It is an important section that must be written after a thorough search and understanding of the collected literature. This section covers the core content of the monograph. Cover more than 50% of the total monograph in this section. Write the summary of each trial or very important trials. If too many trials are available, make a careful selection of the trials based on the strength of evidence of the available clinical trials. As far as possible, segregate the trials logically, arrange and support them with appropriate graphs and tables. You can expect most of the corrections in this section from the client.

Indications: Write both labeled as well as off-label indications. The client's product positioning or their medicolegal affairs department will suggest the drug indications. Sometimes, off-label indications are also covered.

Safety and tolerability: Elaborate this section highlighting the trials on the safety and tolerability. Otherwise, the safety and tolerability data from the efficacy trials are sufficient. To avoid data repetition and redundancy, use tables and graphs to summarize the data. Bring out points that are in favor of the molecule, thereby highlighting its better safety profile when compared to other competitor drug or class of drugs.

Dosage and administration: Give the approved dosage and routes of administration of the drug. Discuss administration methods in detail, especially if the route of administration is intravenous/subcutaneous/ intramuscular. Write succinctly, the method of reconstitution and dilution.

Conclusion/Summary: Write a complete overview of the product monograph, preferably in bullet points. We would consider it as a quick review guide, wherein it should help the doctors to get the gist of the monograph in quick time.

References: The credibility of the monograph depends on the references cited. Published and authentic evidences should adequately support all sections.

Chapter - 20

Detail Aid or Visual Aid

Detail aid or sales aid or visual aid is a print piece (booklet or brochure or flipchart) or an electronic document containing product information. Pharmaceutical sales representatives use the detail aid (print or in eDetailing programs) to engage physicians in a productive dialog about a drug in the name of brand. The detail aid is primarily a marketing tool that incorporates creative elements such as photos, slogans, and brand logos. Importance is given to the brand than to the original molecule. The input is pictorial with graphs and tables that are self-explanatory. There is more scope for creativity. Each page in a detail aid is based on concepts. Medical representatives would get less than 5 min to explain about the brand and therefore, flipchart should be crisp and visually eye-catching.

Flipcharts are the age-old format of visual aids, which the medical representatives used to carry in their bags. Now days, these hard bound flipcharts are being replaced by eDetail aid. The purpose of eDetails is the same as the flipcharts, except that they are designed in an interactive format. eDetail aids are specifically designed for tabs/ipads. It can be as simple as a powerpoint presentation or sophisticated film with good interactive platform. The advantage of eDetail aid is the convenience of using 2D or 3D animations, or short films with or without a voice over. Use of interactive tools enables one to simplify complex data in an interesting manner. The aesthetics of presentation matters the most as the doctors would remember a well presented eDetail.

20.1   Writing a Detail Aid or Visual Aid

The detail aids are used for launching/re-launching a product, new indications and brand extensions/new formulations. The detail-aid has less text, more pictures and graph. The USP of the brand is the appropriately highlighted.

In case of brand launch, the storyline of a detail aid is similar to a product monograph, except that it is concept-based and more pictorial in nature. The content of a detail aid typically includes brand/drug's efficacy, clinical data in support of the manufacturer's claims, charts and graphs, guidance for dosing and administration of the drug, and product's tolerability and safety. It may also include the official labeling.

Although the content will be scientific, it has to be developed based on a concept, which would tell a story. The clinical data should be blended along with a concept and appropriate graphics. Usually the first one or two pages would describe a problem and then the next couple of them would introduce the brand, its indications along with its USPs. In the subsequent pages, each indication /USPs will be described in a line or two, which has to be supported by a graph or suitable image (concept-based). Every page content must be simple and contain only one message. The numerical data supporting the claim should be presented as graphs or tables. The graphical representation of data should be simple and without any ambiguity. Wherever, there is relevant competition, comparative data can be depicted with authentic reference back-up. Each of the pages should be supported by proper scientific references.

20.2　Writing an eDetail Aid

The content writing is the same as writing a print detail aid, except that one has to develop a visual or written storyboard for creating the eDetail aid. The medical writers have to coordinate with digital graphic designers, animators, voiceover artists and IT team.

Chapter - 21

Symposium Highlights

Another part of the marketing strategy is to invite experts from across the world to deliver a talk. Experts would have worked extensively in the respective field or would have been the principal investigator or part of a large trial. Experts usually share their experiences with Indian doctors. Pharma industries organize a symposium in 3–4 cities, where discussion or Q & A will follow the presentation by the expert. Practically, very few doctors get to attend the symposium and benefit from the direct interaction. Presentations by internationally renowned speakers are available to watch online or to read booklets on the symposium.

The purpose here is to reach a wider audience who were not able to attend the conference/symposium. For the benefit of other doctors, deliverables based on the symposium are circulated to other doctors as a part of promotional strategy. The deliverables include an interactive compact disc (CD) of the presentation and discussion; symposium highlight bulletin, scientific booklet and Q & A brochure. The output also serves as a key message reminder for those who attended the meeting. You can reach a far larger audience when you present highlights of proceedings.

Concrete summary is the first thing participants look for when they attend a successful conference. The most important tool you can give them is a timely, reliable summary that helps them do something with what they have learned. Initially, you will be provided with audio/video and slide decks of the presentation. The audio/video tape is usually sent for transcription, if symposium highlights are required in printed form.

21.1 Interactive CD

For the interactive CD, improvement in the audio and editing of the original audio/video track is necessary to make the presentation more aesthetic. The presentation is either presented in one stretch or broken into subsections (based on the outline that we deduce out of the presentation). We can have the option of auto run of the whole presentation or the user can make his choice in viewing any of the subsection of the presentation. The speaker's audio/video is synchronized with the slides. At times, the transcript of the speech itself can be provided in the same window. For the discussion or Q & A section, answers to each of the question is synchronized with the video. The Q & A can be categorized according to the places where the symposiums were held.

For the development of the CD,

- Provide a clear outline for breaking the video into sections and subsections. Note the start and the stop time for each of the subsections

- Provide the questions

- Once the CD is developed, check the content thoroughly for any mismatch of the audio and the video

- Ensure that all the disclaimers are appropriately placed

21.2   Scientific Booklet

The number of pages usually depend on the length of the presentation. Once you are familiar with the subject that the expert is talking about, you will be able to develop an outline and summarize the talk in presentable manner. You will be able to relate to the thoughts and objective of the speaker. Usually, the presentation will be colloquial and for developing the booklet, we have to alter the language that appeals to the reader. At times, we might have to change the order of the flow to simplify the contents and remove any confusion.

The scientific booklet should be written without altering the essence of the presentation. At times, when the speaker does not give the copyrights of the slide deck, then the scientific booklet is developed based on the references cited in the slide decks. Here one has to be careful in picking the data that was discussed by the speaker. The common problem faced by us in this type of project is the phonation/pronunciation of certain terms. This can be overcome by carefully observing the slides and the transcript. At times, there are chances for errors in the transcript (transcripts are usually not error-proof, unless it is done by a professional). You need to appropriately correct the spell errors by crosschecking the terms/terminology with respect to the subject. (For e.g., The transcript had 'tunicate' instead of 'tourniquet'. The subject was orthopedic surgery-related so we had to correct the error).

- For the development of scientific booklet, First, go through the slides and make yourself comfortable with the flow
- Hear/view to the audio/video in conjunction with the slides once or twice
- If you find it difficult to understand, then listen once again and use the transcript to help you with diff cult terms or speaker's pronunciation
- Then develop the content outline for the booklet
- Recreate the slides to match the layout design of the booklet
- Write the content in a manner you write any article but here you are guided by the speaker's transcript and slides
- Use the reference provided in the slide for writing a better content
- Intersperse the contents with important slides but sometimes, the client would insist having the complete set of slides in the booklet
- Eliminate the pronouns
- With respect to the discussion or Q & A session, edit the transcript and present it concisely without any grammatical and technical errors

21.3 Highlight Bulletin

Highlight bulletin is usually a 4-page brochure, which usually provides an overview of the symposium. A journalist attending the symposium submits it like a news report.

21.4 Q & A Booklet

This is interaction or the discussion part that takes place after every symposium or conference. The views and counterviews, questions and answers (by the speaker) are refined into a readable format for the benefit of all others who did not have a chance to attend the symposium or conference. The Q & A sessions provide practical clues and add value to the clinician, so every question and answer should be carefully reviewed and written.

Chapter - 22

Advisory Board Meetings

Experts in a particular therapeutic area meet regularly and take the initiative of formulating a guideline. When there is no evidence-based data to guide the clinicians, such expert meetings/advisory board meetings are conducted to formulate a consensus statement or guideline for a particular guideline. Experts share their clinical experiences through presentations related to a pre-decided topic. After the presentation, experts engage in elaborate discussions. Based on the available level of evidences, experts voice their consent through voting. Subsequently, the members formulate, review and circulate the guidelines among the experts for approval. Once the final draft is ready, the experts publish it in journals for the benefit of all other doctors.

As a medical writer, you may be involved in

- the constitution of advisory board
- formulating aims and objectives of the board
- selecting topics for discussion
- coordinating with expert panel
- conducting of advisory board meeting
- generating consensus or reports

Medical writers need to participate during the advisory board proceedings, record and write articles based on the proceedings of the meeting. Writing inputs for advisory board meetings is no different from that of writing of symposium highlights. Generally, you will have to prepare a short executive summary, compile data from the scientific sessions.

Chapter - 23

Brochure

B rochures usually comprise of one topic in detail but succinctly. A latest journal article pertaining to one or more aspect the drug is usually selected for writing a brochure. Otherwise, in a series of brochures, each unique selling potential (USP) of the drug is discussed independently in each issue.

23.1   Writing the Content for Brochure

A brochure ranges from 2 to 6 pages. In a brochure, discuss only one topic. Based on the client's brief, a brochure can be voluminous or sparsely written. The style of writing a brochure ranges from writing a review article to a detail aid. It is mandatory to intersperse the content with graphs and tables as designing elements are restricted to front page only.

- Select a catchy title
- Understand the data collected and provided to you
- Prepare a content outline
- In the introduction, focus on the USP that you are going to discuss further in the article. Provide epidemiology data, pertaining to Indian scenario, if any
- Build the content for the outline. Support it with tables and graphs
- Give highlighting points
- Cite appropriate references

If you are writing a brochure from a single article, use the cross-references to build your own content for introduction, rationale and discussion. By doing this, you will be giving a new look to the article and simplifying the content for the better readability.

Chapter - 24

Newsletters

Newsletters range between 4 and 16 pages. Depending on the number of pages and the client requirement, a newsletter contains two or more of the following sections:

- Short reviews on drug updates/disease updates/diagnostic updates
- Case studies
- Expert opinion
- Guidelines/regulatory news/medico-legal issues
- **Journal scan:** A brief writing on latest research published in journals
- **Conference news:** List of upcoming important conferences
- **Conference updates:** A brief writing on latest papers or posters presented in conferences
- **Book reviews:** Writing reviews on the recently published medical books
- **Quiz/crosswords:** Multiple choice questions/picture quiz/ crossword puzzles/word jumble
- **Non-medical:** Jokes/quiz/travel/cooking/etc

Short reviews are written typically in a manner any medicomarketing article is written. An interesting case study obtained from leading practitioners is presented along with a discussion that is usually in favor of the drug promoted by the client. At times, instead of case study, an expert's interview or his opinion on a drug/disease/diagnosis is published. New therapeutic guideline from different associations is written. Regulatory news on new indications/new approvals/brand extensions/ warnings and precautions are provided.

Chapter - 25

Pharmaceutical Brand Website

In this electronic age, hosting a brand website has become one of the modes of marketing for pharma companies. Each company would develop a brand website with varying objectives. The design and content of the website would depend on the objective of promotion.

25.1   Objective of Website

The key objective of brand websites could be centered on any of the following themes.

- To create brand awareness
- To provide scientific updates related to the disease
- To promote brand role in disease management
- To promote key messages of the brand
- To provide general information to patients
- Build image of the pharma company as a company that understands healthcare professionals

25.2   Target Audience

The readers of the website could be doctors, patients and caregivers or all of them. Therefore, the content and the complexity of content provided in the website depend on the target audience.

25.3   Process of Developing a Website

The process of developing of website involves the following step.

- Domain name selection

- Hosting of website
- Writing contents
  - ➢ Phase 1 – static content
  - ➢ Phase 2 – dynamic content
- Designing
- Annual maintenance
- Measuring the success of website
- Traffic/Visitors
- Engagement (Sign up) tools used – discussion forum, newsletters

25.4 Standard Content in a Webpage

The usual website contains the following sections
- Home
- About the website
- For healthcare professionals
  - ➢ Articles pertaining to disease management
  - ➢ Case studies
  - ➢ Video interviews of experts
  - ➢ Guidelines
  - ➢ Non-medical information for doctors
  - ➢ Useful links for doctors like journals, associations, conference websites
- For patients
  - ➢ Basic information about disease
  - ➢ Tips on coping with the disease
  - ➢ Managing adverse effects of drugs
  - ➢ Patient forums
  - ➢ Ask the expert
- Contact
- Legal disclaimer
- Logos

25.5 Writing Content for Websites

First, it is important to know the objective of the brand website. Based on the objective, initially, the static content is written. Then depending on the periodicity of the content, the relevant dynamic content is written. The length of articles written for a website should be less than 500 words or depending on the webpage design (up to three scrolls). The language should be simple, engaging and supported by relevant images. Content and images used for website should not violate the copyrights. Appropriate references should be cited and permission to reproduce partial or full content/image should be obtained from the owners.

Chapter - 26

Content for Social Media

Social media such as Facebook, Twitter and YouTube are used to engage with consumers or patients on healthcare-related topics. Increasing number of patients are turning to social media to learn more about their disease and treatments as most of the information they receive from traditional sources is difficult to understand and interpret. Pharmaceutical companies are increasingly using of social media to promote disease information to doctors or to patients; however, no direct brand promotion will be done through social media.

26.1 Writing Content for Social Media

Writing content for social media is interesting and creative. The content is usually one line and wherever possible, an interesting image or concept can be used. The content can be provided as an URL that links to an article from another website. Most often, the content would have to be added on a daily basis and so there should be a variety in writing the content. The information should be up-to-date and relevant to the context of promotion.

Chapter - 27

Patient Education Materials

A well-informed patient will be able to better comprehend the course of disease and its management. Patient education inputs are intended for

- Educating patients and/or their caretakers
- Helping patients to maintain or to improve their health

An informed and educated patient can participate in their own treatment, improve outcomes, help identify errors before they occur, and reduce their length of stay. Other benefits of patient education include the following:

- Increase the patients' ability to deal with and manage their health
- Assist the patients' and their caretakers in understanding the prevailing health status, treatment options, and consequences of disease management
- Support patients to make decision on their health
- Increases the probability of patients to follow a healthcare plan
- Increase patients confidence in their self-care
- Reduce treatment complications
- Better treatment compliance through effective communication and patient education
- Help patients to build trust and rapport with the doctor
- Goodwill from the doctor to the patients and their caretakers

The various patient education inputs include:

- Piano folder
- Booklets
- Posters
- Tear-offs

27.1 Writing Content for Patient Education Inputs

Usually, the content for patient education would be about the disease and its management. In addition, there will be a section on DO's and DON'Ts. A patient or a caretaker reading patient education material should know the answers for the following questions.

1. What is the disease or disorder?
2. What are the signs and symptoms?
3. What is the cause?
4. What are the risk factors? or Who are at risk of developing the disease or disorder?
5. How is the disease or disorder diagnosed? What is the laboratory and other tests recommended?
6. What are the treatment options?
7. What are the lifestyle and home remedies?
8. What are the preventive measures?
9. DO's and DON'Ts

First of all, determine the target audience and objectives

- Who will read your health materials?
- What is the age group?
- What do you want your target audience to do as a result of reading your document?

Language has to be as simple as possible and easy to understand. Structure the material logically. Use active voice verbs, not passive. Write using a conversational, rather than a stiff, formal, clinical tone. Weed out unnecessary information. Include only information that is relevant to the objectives of that particular document. Use alternative words for complex words, medical jargon, abbreviations, and acronyms. Be consistent with terms. For example, don't use "drugs" and "medications" interchangeably in the same document. Emphasize the benefits of the desired behavior. Use bullets wherever possible. Use question and answer format to pull them into reading. Use authentic sources for patient education.

The following websites and journals are useful in preparing the patient education materials.

1. Mayo Clinic: http://www.mayoclinic.com
2. National Institutes of Health (NIH): http://www.nhlbi.nih.gov
3. American Academy of Family Physicians: www.aafp.org
4. Association and society websites

Patient education input is the best way to exhibit your creativity. Pictures and figures should complement the text provided. You should actively work in conjunction with designer to get a better output. Use colors that are appealing to your target audience. Balance the use of text, graphics, and clear or 'white space'. Try for 40–50% white space. Use fonts large enough for your target audience. For a preliminary draft, you can use Google images, but when designing, it is better to use copyright free images or purchase images from image banks. To get a better output, it is good to get an artist to create the relevant images. Few of the image banks are

1. Thinkstock: www.thinkstockphotos.in/
2. Gettyimages: http://www.gettyimages.in/oxfordscientific
3. Sciencephoto: http://www.sciencephoto.com/

PART - IV

Writing Different Types of Articles

Before writing, it is important to know the type of article that you are going to write. Based on the source articles and the required type of input, the different types of articles include

- *Journal and conference news*
- *Journal or a conference scan*
- *Review articles*
- *Case studies*
- *Expert opinion*
- *Guidelines*
- *Book reviews*

Chapter - 28

Journal and Conference News

Journal and conference news provide a brief glimpse on the latest happenings in medicine. This section is usually a part of newsletter, bulletin, or booklet. Sometimes, a newsletter contains only journal scan and conference updates.

28.1 Writing a Journal or a Conference Scan

Journal or conference scan/updates refers to writing news – like an article. The content for this section is based on the recent abstracts or full-text articles from recent journal articles and conference abstracts published in journals or in any of the medical websites (e.g., Medscape). Nevertheless, follow the below steps to write journal scan or conference updates from the abstracts.

1. Select and read the abstracts for writing journal scan
2. Identify and understand the following sections in the abstract:
    (a) What is the context of the study undertaken?
    (b) Who were the study population?
    (c) What was the intervention?
    (d) What was the duration of treatment?
    (e) What is the duration of follow-up?
    (f) What are the primary and secondary outcome measures?
    (g) What is the result?
    (h) What is the author conclusion?
    (i) Is there any clinical implication of the study?
3. Then paraphrase in the following order
    (a) Frame an appropriate title
    (b) Write a line or two substantiating the title

(c) Describe the background or the context (if required)

(d) Write the study method:
  (i) The study design and patient population
  (ii) The treatment given
  (iii) The duration of intervention and the follow-up period.
  (iv) The primary and secondary outcome measures.

(e) Write the results
  (i) Create tables or graphs, if there is a scope

(f) Write the clinical implication or future prospects, if discussed in the original article.

The varieties of inputs that can be developed based on abstracts include:

- Q & A booklets
- Medical newsletters
- Conference news booklets.

Chapter - 29

Review Articles

A review gives an overview of the disease in context to the new diagnostic/therapeutic options or existing therapeutic options. A review article will be a regular type writing for journals and newsletters.

29.1 Writing a Review Article

Review articles are as good as any review article published in the journals, except that it is not peer reviewed. A review article is usually 4-5 pages long. It is a part of any input developed. It is usually based on drug-disease/disorder perspective. Before beginning to write, it is necessary to understand the client's requirement and quickly comprehend the available literature. The best way to do is to go through a latest drug review article published in the journal. Just write a preliminary title to start (you can change to a better one in the end). Next, the content approach should be ready in your mind. Write the content approach first and then look for relevant reference to fill the sections. Estimate the number of pages; decide the length of each section. Remember that your main theme of the article should preferably cover50-60% of your review.

- Write an appropriate title
- Understand the client's brief
- Collect references using the appropriate key words
- Understand the data collected and those provided to you
- Prepare a content outline.
- Write a good introduction
- Build the storyline and support the content with tables and graphs
- Give highlighting points
- Cite appropriate references

Chapter - 30

Case Studies

Doctors publish case studies for sharing unique experiences with fellow doctors. Case studies from key opinion leaders add value to the brand. In case studies, the treatment would ideally comprise the client's molecule; nevertheless, some unique case studies have no relevance to client's molecule.

30.1   Writing Case Studies

Writing case studies is an art. It combines knowledge (theoretical and practical) and writing skills. Initially, doctors provide the case studies in a raw format. Read the case study, and for more information, search the literatures. Exercise caution to avoid any errors of commission or omission. As a medical writer, present the case studies in the following format.

Case presentation: Write the clinical circumstances that lead the patient to the doctor.

Medical and family history: Write about the medical and any significant family history.

Clinical evaluation: Write about physical examination (height, weight, blood pressure, pulse rate, etc), laboratory investigations and other tests performed.

Diagnosis: Write the diagnosis.

Treatment and management: Write about all the treatment and management aspects. Here ensure that the client's molecule is used. Otherwise, confirm with the client or your senior.

Follow-up: Write on the treatment prognosis.

Discussion: Write a very short review article on the disease and treatment. Ensure that the communication is in context to the case presented. Focus on the client's molecule. If there a scope, discuss about the diagnostic and treatment in depth. Support your discussion with appropriate references.

Alternatively, you can present case studies as a narrative. Although the content covers all the above points, the style of writing will be different.

Chapter - 31

Expert Opinion

Although, there are vast data available on the disease and its management, the practical aspect of managing the disease varies from one clinical scenario to another. As an expert in one specialty, the key opinion leader (KOL) is bound to have overcome obstacles and garnered practical knowledge in managing their patients. Very few doctors would have the privilege of directly interacting with the KOL, so experts share their views and provide practical tips to other doctors with respect to the diagnoses, management and treatment.

31.1 Writing Expert Opinion

Expert opinions range from few lines up to a couple of pages. Expert opinion can be a standalone article or a highlighting point for a main article. Expert opinions are value add to the written article. Depending on the type of project, main article can have one or more expert opinion. Each of the expert opinion has the credential of the sharing KOL. Writers usually need not write expert opinions. KOLs themselves write the content for expert opinion. All they have to do is to present the data free from grammatical and technical errors. Avoid any error of commission. Nevertheless, to avoid delay in project delivery, writers write a few lines on the molecule or the drug, and get it endorsed by the KOL. Writing an expert opinion is an art, it comes from experience.

Chapter - 32

Guidelines

S ocieties or group of experts issues guidelines to standardize the diagnoses and treatment modalities. Guidelines are originally published based on evidence or consensus. If a recent guideline, speaks about the clients' molecule then it is logical to highlight the guideline recommendations and update the doctor on the newer guideline. Practically, guidelines are comprehensive and lengthy. For the benefit of doctors, writers have to summarize guidelines.

32.1   Writing Guidelines

Writing guidelines is simple, when understood properly. Depending on the number of pages required, guidelines could be written as short as 1 page and as long as 12 pages. The format for an elaborate guideline can be based on the following lines.

- In the introduction, write about the society or the group of experts and the background for developing the guideline.
- Next give a table for the level and gradation of evidence.
- Write a section on diagnostic recommendation. Support the recommendation with evidence (data discussed in the guideline).
- Write a section on treatment recommendations (all levels of treatment) and support the recommendations with evidence (data discussed in the guideline).
- Highlight the content where the client's molecule is discussed.

For a short guideline, cover the topics exclusively suggested by the client.

Chapter - 33

Book Reviews

A book review is a description and an evaluation on the quality, purpose and usefulness of a book. Book reviews are part of content for a newsletter, to provide variety. It just adds value to the newsletter or a booklet. Sometimes, it is a filler instead of an advertisement.

33.1   How to Write Book Reviews?

To write a book review, you need to read and analyze the contents thoroughly. When you answer the following in paragraphs, it becomes book review.

- Is the book's topic important?
- Is the information timely?
- Is the content appropriate for the intended audience?
- Is the book appropriately organized?
- Is the writing clear?
- Is the style consistent throughout the book?
- Is my favourite topic covered appropriately?
- Has the author included appropriate tables and figures?
- Are there misspellings and minor errors?
- Are there significant errors of fact?
- Is the index adequate to find what I want to find?
- Are the paper and binding of good quality?
- Is the book worth the cost?
- Do you recommend the book and, if so, for which readers?

PART - V

Biostatistics for Medical Writers

Biostatistics is a branch of statistics which facilitates proper interpretation of scientific data that is generated through the clinical trials. Biostatistics is altogether a different subject, nevertheless, it is important for medical writers to be aware of the statistical terms which are intergrate part of results and study design.

Chapter - 34

Essential Biostatistics for Medical Writing

Medical writers should not only have subject knowledge but also understand the data presented in the research paper. A combination of knowledge and research understanding enables them to write better for the right target audiences. For understanding the data, it is important to be aware of certain terminologies found in research papers. Biostatistics is an exclusive subject. It is not mandatory for medical writers to master it; however, a brief idea of the terms used could help writers make the text more meaningful to the readers.

34.1   Prevalence vs. Incidence

'Prevalence' refers to the number of existing cases at the time of counting (i.e., at a given point of time). A cross-sectional study usually gives a count of all the people with illness (prevalence). Prevalence is calculated by dividing the number of persons with the illness at a particular point of time by the number of individuals examined.

'Incidence' refers to the rate of new cases arising. Incidence depicts the rate at which a disease is occurring. It is calculated for a specific time period, usually for one year, by dividing the number of new cases by the size of the population under consideration who are initially disease free or at risk of developing the illness. A longitudinal study usually involves at least two time points and therefore depicts the change in the rate of occurrence of the illness.

Incidence vs. Prevalence

Example 1: Study by Mohan et al. explains the incidence.

The Chennai Urban Population Study (CUPS) is an on-going epidemio logical study conducted in two residential colonies in Chennai. The baseline data were collated between 1996 and 1997. After 8 years of follow-up (Figure 34.1), the overall incidence rate of diabetes was 20.2 per 1000 person years and that of pre-diabetes was 13.1 per 1000 person years among subjects with normal glucose tolerance. Out of 37 subjects, who were pre-diabetic at baseline, 15 (40.5%) developed diabetes with an incidence rate 64.8 per 1000 person years.

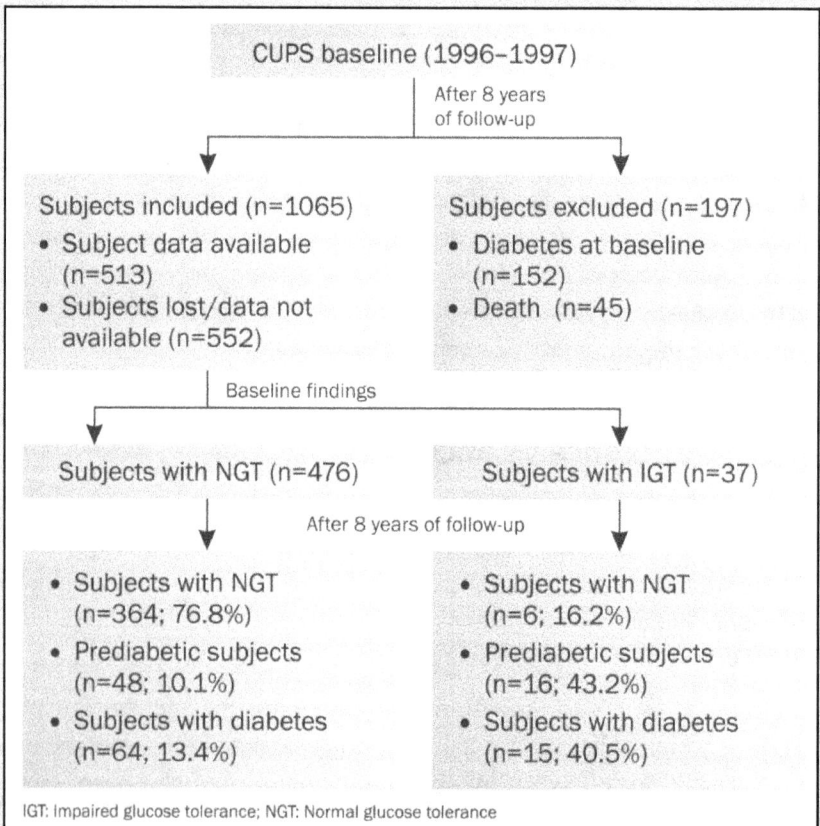

CUPS baseline (1996–1997)

After 8 years of follow-up

Subjects included (n=1065)
- Subject data available (n=513)
- Subjects lost/data not available (n=552)

Subjects excluded (n=197)
- Diabetes at baseline (n=152)
- Death (n=45)

Baseline findings

Subjects with NGT (n=476)

Subjects with IGT (n=37)

After 8 years of follow-up

- Subjects with NGT (n=364; 76.8%)
- Prediabetic subjects (n=48; 10.1%)
- Subjects with diabetes (n=64; 13.4%)

- Subjects with NGT (n=6; 16.2%)
- Prediabetic subjects (n=16; 43.2%)
- Subjects with diabetes (n=15; 40.5%)

IGT: Impaired glucose tolerance; NGT: Normal glucose tolerance

Source: Mohan V, Deepa M, Anjana RM, Lanthorn H, Deepa R. Incidence of diabetes andpre-diabetes in a selected urban south Indian population (CUPS-19). J Assoc Physicians India. 2008;56:152–157

Figure 34.1: Baseline and follow-up status of study population

Example 2: Ramachandran et al. report on the prevalence of diabetes and impaired glucose tolerance.

Subjects (n = 11216; 5288 men; 5928 women) aged ≥20 years, representing all socio-economic strata were randomly selected and subjected to oral glucose tolerance test (OGTT). Prevalence of diabetes and impaired glucose tolerance were 12.1% and 14.0% respectively, with no gender differences. Subjects aged <40 years had a higher prevalence of impaired glucose tolerance than diabetes (12.8% vs. 4.6%, p < 0.0001). This national study demonstrated that the prevalence of diabetes was high in urban India.

Source: Ramachandran A, Snehalatha C, Kapur A, et al. High prevalence of diabetes and impaired glucose tolerance in India: National Urban Diabetes Survey. Diabetologia. 2001;44: 1094–1101.

The prevalence data associates the illness to a particular risk factor while the incidence data provides information beyond the association of the illness to the causation.

34.2   Probability

Probability is a measure of the chance of obtaining a desired outcome from an event. The probability of the occurrence of an event is measured between 0 and 1. Probability of an event or illness = number of outcomes that favor an event or illness/total number of possible outcomes.

Probability

Example 1: What is the probability of getting an even number when you roll a dice?
  • Total number of possible outcomes = 6 (1 or 2 or 3 or 4 or 5 or 6)
  • Total number of outcomes favoring the event 'an even number'
        = 3 (i.e., 2 or 4 or 6)
  • So the probability of getting an desired outcome (even number)
        = 3 ÷ 6 = 0.5

Example 2: What is the probability of being affected by swine flu?
In a class of 30 children, if the probability of being affected by swine flu (an event that occurs) is equal to one, then all 30 children will suffer from swine flu. On the contrary, if the probability is zero, then no children will suffer from swine flu. If the chance of being affected by swine flu is as good as not getting swine flu, then the probability of getting swine flu is ½ or 0.5 (i.e., 50%). If the probability of getting swine flu is P, then the probability of children not getting swine flu is (1 − P).

34.3 Measures of Effect Size

Odds ratio, relative risk reduction, absolute risk reduction, and the number needed to treat (NNT) to prevent a bad outcome are the commonly used measures of effect size. Follow the example given under each section to understand each of the measures of effect size.

34.3.1 Odds Ratios

Odds ratios are used in case-control studies to assess the occurrence of an outcome in the presence of a certain factor. It describes the probability of an event occurring in the presence of a factor (or exposure) and in the absence of a factor (exposure). Odds ratio is a simple ratio that depicts the odds of an event occurring in the exposed group versus the unexposed group.

Case-control studies (prospective or retrospective) analyze the data to establish the strength of the factors that appear to be associated with the outcome. Odds ratio is used to estimate the strength of association of the variable with the outcome of interest. However, one cannot calculate risk in a case-control study.

Odds ratios

Example 1: What are the odds of suffering from CAD when one had diabetes or hypertension?

Table 34.1: Data obtained for the total female population
[N=198; 100 (Control) + 98 (CAD patients)]

Risks (Total number of patients)	Patients with CAD
Diabetes mellitus (94)	62
Family H/O IHD (15)	33
Hyperlipidemia (102)	57
Hypertension (66)	36

Diabetes as risk factor: Let us calculate the impact of diabetes on CAD (i.e., the odds ratio for diabetes as a risk factor for CAD). From Table 34.1, the following matrix can be deduced.

	CAD	No. CAD (control)	Total
Female patients with diabetes	62	32	94
Female patients without diabetes	36	68	104

- In female patients with diabetes, the odds of suffering
  CAD = 62/32 = 1.94.
- In female patients without diabetes, the odds of suffering
  CAD = 36/68 = 0.53
- The odds ratio is 1.94/0.53 = 3.66.

Hypertension as risk factor: In a similar fashion, let us calculate the impact of hypertension on CAD. From Table 34.1, the following matrix can be deduced.

	CAD	No CAD (control)	Total
Female patients with hypertension	36	30	68
Female patients without hypertension	62	70	132

- In female patients with hypertension, the odds of suffering CAD = 36/30 = 1.2.
- In female patients without hypertension, the odds of suffering CAD=62/70=0.8.
- The odds ratio is 1.2/0.89 = 1.34

Hence, diabetes is a strong risk factor for CAD compared to hypertension.

Source: Nazeer M, Naveed T, AmanUllah. A case—control study of risk factors for coronary artery disease in Pakistani females. Annals. 2010;16(3):162–168.

- An odds ratio of 1 suggests that the event is equally likely in both groups
- An odds ratio greater than one implies that the event is more likely in the first group.
- An odds ratio less than one implies that the event is less likely in the first group

34.3.2 Relative Risk Reduction/Absolute Risk Reduction /NNT

Relative risk reduction is the difference between the event rates in relative terms. Absolute risk reduction (also called the risk difference) is the simple difference in the event rates between the two arms of treatment. Relative risk reduction is often more impressive than absolute risk reduction. Absolute risk reduction reduces as the event rates reduce, while the relative risk reduction remains constant. The number of patients who would have to receive the treatment for 1 of them to benefit is NNT. It is calculated as 100 divided by the absolute risk reduction expressed as a percentage (or 1 divided by the absolute risk reduction expressed as a proportion).

Relative Risk Reduction/Absolute Risk Reduction/NNT

Example 1: Deducing the relative risk reduction/absolute risk reduction/NNT.

Initially, 20,536 patients were randomized to simvastatin (n = 10269) or placebo (n = 10,267). At the end of the study, 10,232 in the simvastatin and 10,237 in the placebo group were eligible for analysis. All-cause mortality rates in the simvastatin and placebo groups were 1328 and 1507, respectively. Treatment with simvastatin reduced relative risk of death by 12.2% (see below for calculation).

The following matrix was deduced from the given data.

Treatment	Total patients	No. of patients who died	No. of patients who survived
Simvastatin	10.232	1328	8904
Placebo	10,237	1507	8730

Risk of death with simvastatin = 1328/10232 = 0.129 or 12.9% = (x)

Risk of death with placebo = 1507/10237 = 0.147 or 14.7% = (y)

Relative risk (risk ratio) of death with simvastatin = 0.129/0.147 = 0.878 or 87.8% (x/y)

Relative risk reduction (number of deaths reduced with simvastatin treatment) = 100% - 87.8% = 12.2% = (1 - x/y) × 100

Absolute risk reduction = |12.9-14.7| = 1.8%

Number needed to treat (NNT) =1/1.8 = 55.5 (55.5 patients have to take statins to prevent 1 death among them).

Source: Heart Protection Study Collaborative Group. MRC/BHF Heart Protection Study of cholesterol lowering with simvastatin in 20536 high-risk individuals: A randomised placebo controlled trial. Lancet. 2002;360:7–22.

34.3.3 Hazard Ratio

A hazard ratio expresses the effect of a risk factor or exposure on the study outcome, when time to event or survival analyses is used. Hazard ratio is the probability that a patient under observation has an event at that given time. Ratio of hazard rates for each group (i.e., Outcome rate with treatment/Outcome rate without treatment).

Hazard rate for Group 1 at a given timepoint = number of events in group 1/total number of events

Hazard rate for Group 2 at a given timepoint = number of events in group 2/total number of events

Hazard ratio at a given timepoint = Hazard rate for Group 1/Hazard rate for Group 2

- If hazard ratio at a given timepoint = 1, then it means that both groups have equal risks or that the treatment produced no effects.
- If hazard ratio at a given timepoint >1, then there is an increased risk for the event to happen in Group 1.
- If hazard ratio at a given timepoint <1, then there is a decreased risk for the event to happen in Group 1.

Higher the hazard ratio, the greater is the chance that the endpoint will occur sooner in the treated patient than in the control group.

If hazard ratio at a given timepoint = 2, then it implies that at any given time, twice as many patients in the active treatment group are having an event when compared with the comparator group. Please note that a hazard ratio of 2 does not mean that the median survival time is doubled (or halved).

Hazard Ratio

Example 1: Calculating the hazard ratio

Yusuf et al. conducted a multicenter trial involving 20,332 patients who recently had an ischemic stroke. These patients were randomly assigned to telmisartan (80 mg daily; n = 10,146) or placebo (n = 10,186). During a mean follow-up of 2.5 years, a total of 880 patients (8.7%) in the telmisartan group and 934 patients (9.2%) in the placebo group had a subsequent stroke (hazard ratio in the telmisartan group: 0.95; 95% confidence interval [CI]: 0.86 to 1.04; p = 0.23). Major cardiovascular events occurred in 1367 patients (13.5%) in the telmisartan group and 1463 patients (14.4%) in the placebo group (hazard ratio: 0.94; 95% CI: 0.87 to 1.01; p = 0.11). For the calculation of hazard ratio, see below. The following matrix can be deduced from the given data.

Treatment	Patients	Number of patients suffering a subsequent stroke	Number of patients not suffering a subsequent stroke
Telmisartan	10,146	880	9266
Placebo	10,186	934	9252
Total	20,332	1814	18518

Hazard rate for telmisartan: 880/1814 = 0.485

Hazard rate for placebo: 934/1814 = 0.514

Hazard ratio for telmisartan for subsequent incidence of stroke

= 0.485/0.514 = 0.943

Treatment	Patients	Major cardio-vascular events(number of patients	No major cardio-vascular events (number of patients)
Telmisartan	10,146	1367	8779
Placebo	10,186	1463	8723
Total	20,332	2830	17502

Hazard rate for telmisartan: 1367/2830 = 0.483

Hazard rate for placebo: 1463/2830 = 0.516

Hazard ratio for telmisartan for subsequent incidence of major cardiovascular events = 0.485/0.514 = 0.936

Source: Yusuf S, Diener HC, Sacco RL et al. For PRoFESS Study Group. Telmisartan to prevent recurrent stroke and cardiovascular events. N Engl J Med. 2008 Sep 18;359(12):1225–1237.

Hazard ratio can be better understood with this example. Suppose 100 patients are treated for an ailment, and in the first month 2 die; then the hazard rate for Month 1 is 2/100. If 4 people die in the second month, then the hazard ratio for Month 2 is 4/98. Similarly, the hazard rate can be calculated for the placebo and control groups. The ratio of the hazard rates can be calculated at different time points.

34.3.4 Survival Analysis (Time-to-event Analysis)

Survival analysis describes how many people can reach a certain endpoint in time without experiencing a hazard or event other than death. Kaplan Meier is the usual technique performed to analyse survival-time data (i.e., to measure the fraction of subjects living for a certain amount of time after treatment). While analyzing survival data, two functions that are dependent on time are of particular interest: the survival function and the hazard function. The survival function S(t) is defined as the probability of surviving at least to time 't'. The hazard function h(t) is the conditional probability of dying at time 't' having survived to that time.

34.4 Null Hypothesis/Alternate Hypothesis

The null hypothesis simply states that there is no difference between the groups. Alternate hypothesis states that there is a difference between the groups.

34.5 Tests of Significance (p value)

p values of <0.05 are often accepted as 'statistically significant' in medical literature by researchers. A p<0.05 means that result from 5 of 100 experiments appear significant just by chance. Smaller p values indicate stronger evidence against the null hypothesis. p values give no indication about the clinical importance of the observed association.

34.6 Confidence Interval

The technical term for this process of estimating confidence interval is statistical inference. When the outcome of a study is to be extrapolated to the general population (of course provided that the sample is truly representative of the population) then the outcome will fall within some range of sample outcome (plus or minus [±]). To express the extent to which the range is valid, researchers choose 95%, 99%, or 90% confidence levels. Statisticians say that a confidence interval represents a plausible range of values for the true (population) value. Confidence interval is preferred to p values because it depicts the range of possible effect sizes. A meaningful clinical significance can be derived from the size of the effect desired in the study.

- In any study, the width of a confidence interval gives the precision of the estimate. The larger the sample, the narrower and thus more precise is the confidence interval.
- A wide confidence interval may be statistically significant, but not clinically significant. In addition, a wide confidence interval suggests that the sample size is small.
- Confidence interval is calculated for differences in means, proportions, and medians.
  - ➢ If a confidence interval denoting a mean contains 0, then it is not significant.
  - ➢ If a confidence interval denoting a ratio contains 1, then it is not significant.
- **95% confidence interval:** There is a probability of 0.95 that an event/illness will occur within two standard errors of the population mean.

34.6.1 Confidence Intervals for Odds Ratios

If confidence interval for an odds ratio contains 1, then the factor concerned plays no significant role; if confidence interval for an odds ratio does not contain 1, then the concerned factor is a significant risk (or benefit).

34.6.2 Confidence Intervals for Risk Ratios (Relative Risk)

If the confidence interval contains 1, then there is no statistically significant risk associated with the factor involved. If the confidence interval does not contain 1, then the risk ratio is significant; if less than 1, it is 'beneficial', if greater than 1, there is an adverse effect.

34.6.3 Confidence Intervals for Hazard Ratio

Similar to that of odds and risk ratios, if the interval contains 1, the factor is not a statistically significant risk. If it does not contain 1, the factor is a statistically significant risk. Values greater than 1 indicate that the factor increases the risk of death (or the specified clinical outcome), values less than 1 indicate that the factor decreases this risk.

Confidence Intervals for Odds Ratios

Example 1: In the table below, except for hypertension and hyperlipidemia, all other risk factors significantly influence CAD

Table 34.4: Association of risk factors with coronary artery disease in total female population (n = 198)

Variable (H)	CAD (n)	OR (95% CI)	P	Odds ratio (98% CI)
Diabetes mellitus (94)	62	3.65 (2.0-6.5)	<0.00001	
Family H/OIHD (15)	57	2.11 (1.2-3.8)	0.01	
Waist circumference (">35 cm")	57	2.11 (1.2-3.8)	0.01	
Hyperlipedemia	57	1.7 (1.0 – 2.9)	0.08	
Hypertension(66)	36	1.3 (0.7-2.4)	0.3	
				0.5 1 2 3 4 5

Source: Nazeer M, Naveed T, AmanUllah. A case-control study of risk factors for coronary artery disease in Pakistani females. Annals. 2010;16(3):162-168.

Confidence Intervals for Risk Ratios (Relative Risk)

Example 1: A study showing the confidence intervals for risk ratios (relative risk)

Treatment with simvastatin and placebo resulted in 12.9 and 14.7% death; the relative risk of death was 0.87 (0.81-0.94) p = 0.0003. The confidence interval does not contain 1 and therefore, the outcome was significant with a 12.2% relative risk reduction in mortality.

Source: Heart Protection Study Collaborative Group. MRC/BHF Heart Protection Study of cholesterol lowering with simvastatin in 20536 high-risk individuals: A randomised placebo controlled trial. Lancet. 2002; 360:7–22.

Confidence Intervals for Hazard Ratios

Example 1: Observe the study data below for confidence interval for hazard ratio.

Study data		
Total number of patients		20,332
Treatment	Telmisartan	Placebo
Number of patients	10,146	10,186
Total number of stroke	1814	
Number of patients suffering a stroke (%)	880 (8.7%)	934 (9.2%)
Hazard ratio in the telmisartan group for stroke incidence	0.95; 95% confidence interval:0.87 to 1.01; p = 0.11	
Total patients having major cardiovascular event (within6 months of randomization)	2830	
Patients having major cardio-vascular events (within 6 months of randomization) (%)	1367 13.5%)	1463 (14.4%)
Hazard ratio	0.94; 95% CI: 0.87 to 1.01; p = 0.11	
Patients having major cardiovascular events after6 months of treatment (%)	893 (8.8%)	1030 (10.1%)
Hazard ratio	0.87; 95% CI: 0.80 to 0.95; p = 0.004	

From this study, it is evident that telmisartan has no stroke protective effect because the confidence interval for the hazard ratio contains 1 (Hazard ratio: 0.95; 95% CI: 0.87 to 1.01). So, there is no difference between telmisartan and placebo. Similarly, the incidence of major cardiovascular events (within 6 months of randomization) does not favour telmisartan (confidence interval for the hazard ratio contains 1; Hazard ratio: 0.94; 95% CI: 0.87 to 1.01); however, the data for major cardiovascular events after six months of treatment showed that telmisartan was effective in preventing major cardiovascular events after six months of treatment because the confidence interval does not include 1 (0.87; 95% CI: 0.80 to 0.95). Also, note the p value for significance in each of the case.

Source: Yusuf S, Diener HC, Sacco RL, et al. For PRoFESS Study Group. Telmisartan to prevent recurrent stroke and cardiovascular events. N Engl J Med. 2008 Sep 18; 359(12):1225–1237.

34.7 Deducing the Outcome

It is common to observe the terms, 'per-protocol population' or 'intention-to-treat population' in the study methodology or result section. These terms indicate the method by which results are deduced. In non inferiority trials, both intention-to-treat and per-protocol analysis are recommended. Intention-to-treat is the recommended method in superiority trials to avoid any bias.

34.7.1 Per-protocol Analysis

This analysis includes only those subjects who have completed the full course of assigned treatment without any protocol violations. This analysis has greater chances for bias.

34.7.2 Intention-to-treat

Intention-to-treat analysis is a comparison of the treatment groups that includes all patients as originally allocated after randomization. Subjects are analyzed according to the treatment to which they were assigned, regardless of whether they received the treatment or not. This analysis gives a real-time estimate of the benefit of a change in treatment policy rather than of potential benefits in patients who receive treatment exactly as planned.

PART - VI

Beyond Writing

In this section, we share our experience and highlight the other aspects involved in medicomarketing communications.

Chapter - 35

Paper and Printing Process

35.1 Paper Type and Size

You need to know the basics about paper and the printing process so that you can understand and visualize the specifications before writing an article. Two types of papers are commonly used for printing: matte and art paper. Matte paper is not glossy and is easy to read. Art paper is glossy and is used when the look is more important than the content (brochures, visual aids, etc).

Different countries use different paper size standard conventions to express the dimensions of paper (size of paper). The international (International Organization for Standardization [ISO]) paper sizes and the UK metric and imperial sizes (demy, 1/4th demy, 1/8th demy, Crown, 1/2 crown, 1/4th crown, Quarto) are the most commonly used. The international paper sizes are: A, and B series (Figures 35.1 and 35.2). Metric sizes are given in Table 35.1. The amount of text you write in a word file depends on the size of the paper that will be used for the final project. The usual number of pages of content to be written for different sizes of paper is given in Table 35.2.

The quality of the paper is proportional to its thickness. Thickness is expressed as Grams per square meter (GSM). As the GSM increases, the thickness of the paper increases. Thickness varies from 60 GSM (paper user for photocopying) to 210 GSM (paper used for cover pages of books). Depending on the quality, function, and cost of the final product, the thickness of the paper to be used is proposed to the client.

	Width (in mm)	Height (in mm)
A0	841	1189
A1	594	841
A2	420	594
A3	297	420
A4	210	297
Letter	215.9	279.4
Legal	215.9	355.6
A5	148	210
A6	105	148
A7	74	105
A8	52	74

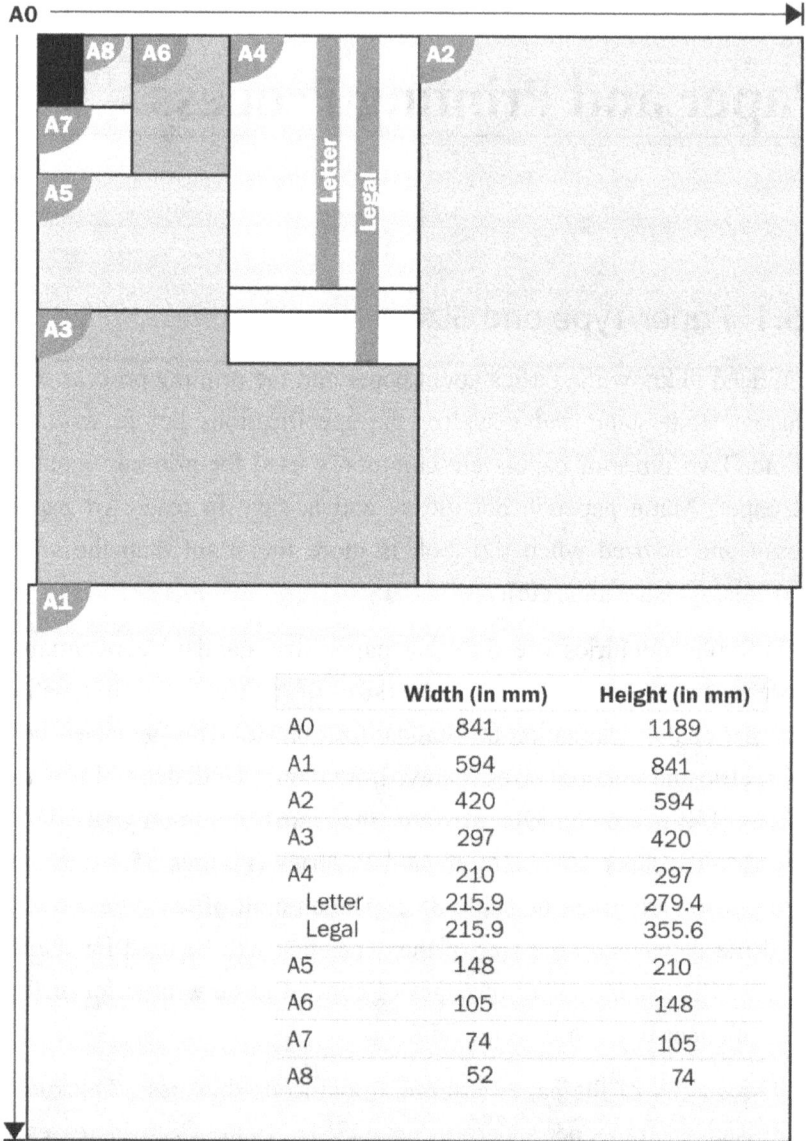

Figure 35.1: Understanding paper sizes of A series

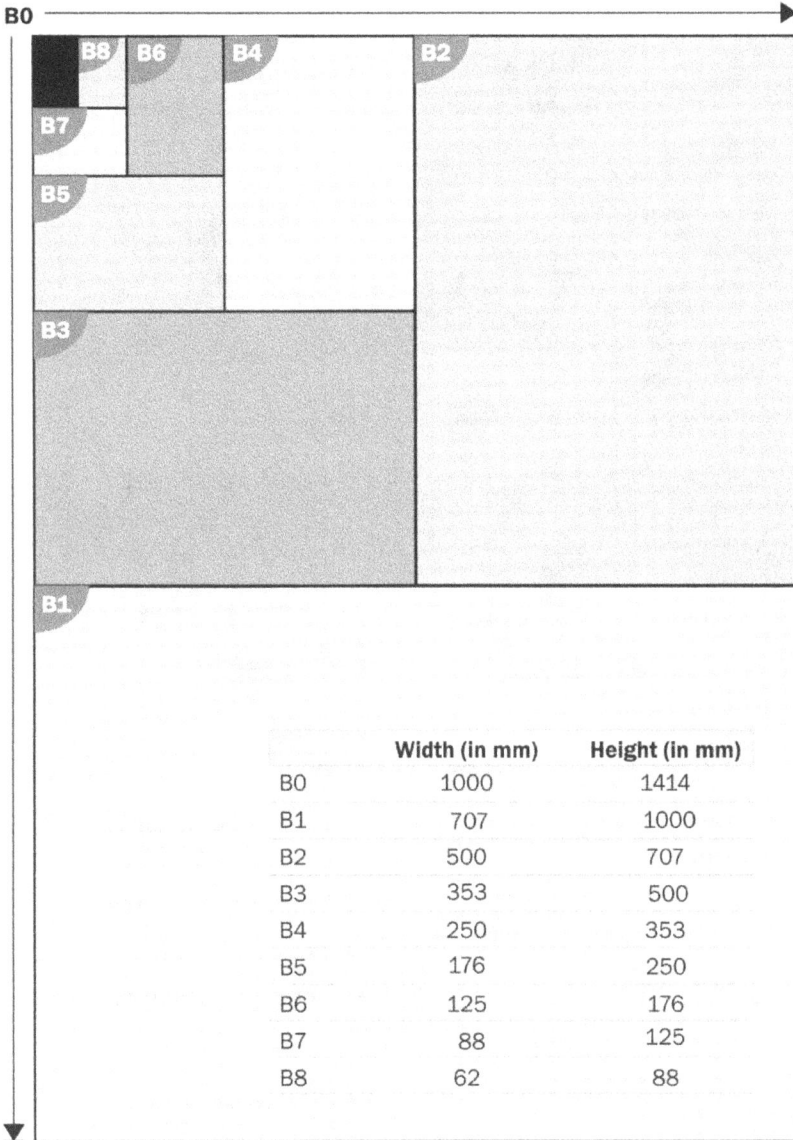

	Width (in mm)	Height (in mm)
B0	1000	1414
B1	707	1000
B2	500	707
B3	353	500
B4	250	353
B5	176	250
B6	125	176
B7	88	125
B8	62	88

Figure 35.2: Understanding paper sizes of B series

Table 35.1: UK metric paper sizes

	Millimeters		Inches		Points	
	Height	Width	Height	Width	Height	Width
Metric Crown Quarto	246	189	9 11/16	7 7/16	697	536
Metric Crown Octavo	186	123	7 5/16	4 13/16	527	349
Metric Large Crown Quarto	258	201	10 3/16	7 7/8	731	570
Metric Large Crown Octavo	198	129	7 13/16	5 1/16	561	366
Metric Demy Quarto	276	219	10 7/8	8 5/8	782	621
Metric Demy Octavo	216	138	8 1/2	5 7/16	612	391
Metric Royal Quarto	312	237	12 1/4	9 5/16	884	672
Metric Royal Octavo	198	129	7 13/16	5 1/16	561	366

35.2 Colors for Offset Printing

1. **Single color**: All text and images will be either in black or any one color

2. **Two-color**: Text and images will be in any 2 colors/mixture of those 2 colors in different proportions.

Table 35.2: Paper size and proportionate number pages of text required in word document

Paper size (for 1 page)	Number of pages in word document with default setting
A2 or ½ demy	2 pages
A4 1/4th demy	1.25
1/4th crown	1
1/8th demy	¾ page

3. **4-color:** Text and images will be in any color. It is called 4-color printing as the four basic colors, cyan, magenta, yellow, and black (CMYK) are used. You can get ANY color by mixing CMYK in different proportions.

4. **Special colors:** Gold, silver and metallic colors are called special colors. Special colours are usually printed separately after 4-color printing. Nowadays, 5-color printing machines are also available.

35.3 Lamination

To protect and change the texture of the paper, the paper is covered with a thin sheet of plastic by applying heat. This process is called lamination. There are several varieties of lamination: gloss, matte, and spot lamination. Spot lamination can be used to highlight a particular area in a figure or an image.

Chapter - 36

Working with Designers

esigners give the final shape to your articles. They make it look attractive to catch the readers' attention. They are an integral part of the medical marketing communication team. Usually designers are graduates in commercial art, while some are DTP (Desktop publishing) operators. Desired qualities in designers include:

- Good design/aesthetic sense
- Proficiency in freehand, illustrator, photoshop, indesign, corel draw, formating or desktop publishing, etc.

They use different softwares to format/design your articles:

1. **Corel draw:** Used for design oriented projects with less number of pages

2. **Page maker/Indesign:** Used to format 12-100 page books with figures and graphs.

3. **Photoshop:** Used to create or edit images

4. **Ventura/Quark express:** Used to format books more than 100 pages

5. **Adobe Illustrator:** It is a vector graphics editor. Adobe Illustrator is the companion product of Adobe Photoshop. Photoshop is primarily meant for digital photo manipulation and photorealistic styles of computer illustration, while Illustrator is used for typesetting and logo graphic areas of design.

Designers will consider brand colors and other specifications (size, number of pages, number of colors, die cut) before starting their design work. Besides the specifications, you would have to give the following details of the project to the designer to get a better output:

- **Drug/Disease background:** psychiatry, cardiology, epilepsy, gynecology, paediatrics, etc.

- **Target group:** Age-wise; men, women, children, or families

- **Kind of images:** Photos, illustrations, vectors, line diagrams, or clipart

- **Overall look:** Positive feel, scientific feel, or human

- Branding guideline

- Earlier design projects (samples) for the same products or brand

Tell your designer what you would like to say through the project rather than how you want it to look. Be clear about the specific features you need. You want your designer to create a design specific to your needs. If you try to add features during the course of time, the design will not fit as well. It is important that you do not tell your designer how to design. Designing might not be your area of expertise. Instead, give the designer your requirements and preferences, and at the same time give them the freedom to create. If you micromanage designers, they may become demotivated and the final output will suffer.

Chapter - 37

Working with Marketing

The marketing team is a vital part of a medical marketing communication company. They are the key players in bringing business. Their primary duty is book orders and act as coordinators between the editorial team and the client. Most of them are life-science graduates with MBA and hence not all of them might be able to comprehend the science part of the content. Nevertheless, it is important to understand each other's roles and communicate effectively for the common benefit.

The key responsibilities of the sales team are:

- To develop business opportunities
- To maintain strong relations with clients
- To provide excellent customer service through continued associations; follow-up on completed projects for client satisfaction and development of further opportunities.

The below mentioned two functions should be very distinct.

- The sales team is responsible for developing opportunities with clients and obtaining signed contracts.
- The editorial and design teams are responsible for delivering those projects.

Overstepping into another department's role and responsibility can lead to 3-way communication with a bigger scope for misunderstanding or misinterpretation. There is no hard-and-fast rule to define the line of communication, but with a standard operating procedure (SOP) in place, embarrassing situations can be avoided.

Sales person can handle minor client queries regarding technical information but it is better to route the major client queries to the editorial, as it would reduce the number of iterations. If clients have a tendency to contact sales after signing of the contract, please explain wherever possible that the outcome of the project is likely to be faster and more efficient through a direct interaction with the editorial/design team. Those working on the project will be able to serve them better to discuss the actual content.

To work as a team, it is important for the members of each team to follow the company's communication protocol. All the communications should be through mail. Compose mails with the utmost respect. Mutual updates of the project status help in planning. In case of difficult situations, a discussion among sales, editorial, and design teams will help to overcome the hurdles. All departments have equal responsibility in successfully delivering a project, and therefore neither should consider themselves superior.

The marketing or sales team and the editorial team will always be at logger-heads almost every day. Nevertheless, it does not mean that it is difficult to run the business. Moreover, none of the situations are difficult to handle.

Marketing Team vs. Editorial Team

Scenario 1: Marketing team complains that editorial never delivers on time.

Editorial teams are usually given project priorities and asked to deliver accordingly. Generally, the team lead will ensure that the projects are delivered on time. Nevertheless, at times, owing to certain issues, the project delivery date is delayed.

- Change in project priorities
- Shortage of writers (owing to leaves or work force attrition)
- Miscalculation of timelines
- Change in project brief after the project has been initiated.

Action plan: In any situation, it is mandatory for the editor or the team lead to immediately inform the marketing about a change in schedule. Otherwise, before changing the priorities, it is better to consult the respective marketing team member and convey the changes. Once it is mutually agreed, the editorial should send a new project delivery timelines to the all the concerned people within the team.

A change in project priorities happens due to change in clients' requirement or billing dates. It is necessary to keep the concerned team members informed about the changes, as early as possible, so that the client are also informed about the change in delivery dates. Never make the mistake of informing the marketing about the delay on the day, the project was initially scheduled for delivery.

Here, open communication among the concerned team members will resolve issues amicably.

Marketing Team vs. Editorial Team

Scenario 2: Marketing team complains that they have received the wrong files that is to be sent for client approval or for print

Quite often or sometimes, the marketing will receive a wrong file from designers or the editorial. The reasons may be

- Wrong file name
- Versions of the correction files not maintained by the designer or editor
- Carelessness on part of designer or editor.
- Too many bounces and big time gap that leads to failure to keep track of the project.

Action plan: Editors and designers should follow a standard pattern of naming files and folders. Every change in the document should be maintained as different versions. Anyone looking into the folder should be able to recognize the latest version and take forward for further action. Every time, before sending a mail, the editors have to counter check the document and ensure that the correct file has been attached.

Here, the person should countercheck before sending the mail. Since, the team lead will be in the mail circuit, it is mandatory for the team lead to open the attachment and check. The marketing should also check the attachment before forwarding it to the client.

Marketing Team vs. Editorial Team

Scenario 3: Client needs reference pack for approval.

It is a cumbersome to arrange reference pack. Nevertheless, it is mandatory for some clients to obtain approval from their medical. Just sending the reference pack might be easy, but sometimes, the clients would need the reference pack with text highlighted.

Action plan: At the time of writing or searching or understanding the project, editors can organise their references in a particular way, that it becomes easy for them to retrieve the references used. Vancouver referencing style gives details of authors' second name, title, journal, date, issue, and page numbers. So, it is better, if the reference pdfs or abstracts are stored with file names depicting the first authors' second name and the year (e.g., Bond J_2013). To avoid a long list of references, the abstracts can be collected separately in a word file. In addition, depending on the client's need, it is better to highlight the texts in the references at the time of resourcing or writing itself

Since, organising a proper reference pack is time consuming; the marketing can quote extra charges for sending the reference pack. In this way, the time spent for organising the reference pack is justified.

Marketing Team vs. Editorial Team

Scenario 4: Client needs formatted copy within a short time after approval of the word copy

Like the editorial, the design team are allotted projects on a daily basis. When there is a scope for sending the designed copies as per client requirement, the editorial and the design will do it. Nevertheless, post formatting, the document should go for a review (quality check of document for recreations of figures, tables, algorithms, etc) and then editors/team leaders approve.

Action plan: Do not delay in scheduling the projects for design. Designers need adequate time to design and format. If the clients request is genuine, then try to re-prioritize the projects in design or involve one more additional designer to complete the project. Always, ensure to explain the client and the marketing about the various steps involved in delivery a quality designed product.

Allocate the work to your ace designer, who is experienced and skilled and is able to deliver a decent product within time constraints. Hurrying projects in design will give way for lot of errors of commission and omission. Once in a way, projects can be hurried through designing, but it should not be a routine affair because over time, the quality of design and the product will suffer.

Marketing Team vs. Editorial Team

Scenario 5: Client complains about the quality of writing.

Quality of writing depends on the editors' experience, skill and attitude. Most of times, the issue with quality writing stems from

- novice writers
- short timelines
- articles outsourced to freelancers owing to lack of in-house manpower
- absence of copyeditor

Action plan: Under any circumstances, the team leader should review the document (according to in-house standards) before it is sent to the client. Extra care should be taken if the article is written by a novice medical writer. As far as possible, do not circumvent the process owing to shortened timelines. It is difficult to control the quality of freelance work, but it is the responsibility of the team lead to review the article before sending it to the client. While planning and giving timeline, keep a day extra as a buffer for reworking or major changes.

Always the team lead or another editor should review the article. In the absence of copyeditor, get the document reviewed by another editor. Have good freelance writers on your list and never try new ones for important projects.

Marketing Team vs. Editorial Team

Scenario 6: The client changes the brief after the first cut

This kind of situation can be expected with one-third of the clients. The problem might be related to a wrong brief or change in the marketing strategy after the project has been initiated.

Action plan: Although the situation will be frustrating, editors have to accept the reality with patience and re-work on the project as a new project. Identify clients who typically change the brief after the first-cut and get approval of the content approach prior to writing. On the other hand, read the initiation mail thoroughly and ask relevant questions before writing.

One-third of the clients might change brief, so it is better to talk frequently to the client to get an insight into his requirements.

Marketing Team vs. Editorial Team

Scenario 7: Change in the product specifications at the time of design or print

There are times, when the specification of the output is changed at the last minute. This usually happens to the carelessness of marketing person while filling the specification column in the initiation mail. Otherwise, the client would change it in the last minute for various reasons. Change of specifications amount to waste of time in developing content and ultimately increases the project cost.

Action plan: Writers are helpless in this situation. They are bound to yield to the requirements. Patience is what required at this time.

Marketing team should understand and appreciate the time involved in developing and designing the content. They should be more careful during initiation of the project. If the change is from the client, then there is nothing one can do other than obliging to the client's need.

Chapter - 38

Working with Clients

In addition to writing, you need to communicate/coordinate with product managers, group product managers, and medical advisors (client). Clients are of different kinds, but each of them would fall into any one of the following categories.

38.1   The Good Perfectionists

These clients know the subject and their brand very well. They are organized and are perfectionists. They know all the references available related to their brand. They know what they want. Such clients expect you to write the best possible article for their product. They push you towards excellence. They are demanding and it is often difficult to meet their expectations. However, once we understand and deliver articles of the right quality, the number of bounces will reduce. These types of clients will give correct feedback on your writing skills and you should take them into consideration. They will help you to set higher standards in writing.

38.2   The Bad-Half-baked

These clients have some knowledge about their brands. They do not know what they want, so their brief would usually be incomplete and they would end up asking for something different. They often fail to plan. They may even change the topic of the project after they see the first draft because they would have clarity in what they want only after seeing the first draft. It is rather frustrating at times to work with such clients.

38.3 The Ugly-Dumb

These clients want an input for distribution. They usually do not know the references available on their brands. They are not bothered about the quality of the content you provide. The design should be impressive, and the content should be less (they do not appreciate going through lengthy articles). They set low standards for writing. If you have many clients who fall into this category, you may develop a false sense of success as a medical writer. It is easy to complete projects for such clients, but they are unhealthy for long-term success in medical writing.

Chapter - 39

Working as a Freelancer

Peeople who need regular income and who are risk-averse should not opt to become a freelancer. Freelancing is suitable for those who are financially stable or those who need extra earnings, besides their regular salary. It is suitable for those who want to work from home. Freelancers have the independence of working at their convenience and timings.

Freelance work is not as easy as it is usually perceived. Freelance work always comes with a tight deadline. As a freelancer, one has to market their own skills and aggressively persue to get projects and remunerations on time. One has to be self-organized, self-motivated, and smart. You will have to take-up various roles: marketing, managing, writing, copyediting, and account keeping. You would have to be committed to deliver quality projects as agreed with the client. Unlike full-time work, you will not have any safety nets to help you deliver better.

39.1   Training

Many freelancers often write, based on their intuition. As a freelancer, you will not be given a second chance to write better. Your exposure to learn from others/peers is limited. Therefore, get trained to improve your quality of writing, and turnaround time. Training will expose you to writing different kinds of projects. Be proficient in MS Word, Excel, and PowerPoint.

39.2 Marketing

It is generally difficult to get your first project. Build a network to market your skills. Circulate your portfolio of projects/deliverables that you can write along with your resume when you pitch for projects. Create a good profile in networking websites such as LinkedIn. Identify and establish contacts with product managers of pharma companies, other medical writers, and managers of healthcare communication companies. There are a number of websites, where you can enlist your services. Be prepared to write a sample project.

39.3 Managing

Be professional in your approach. Confirm the project with appropriate terms and conditions. Save the files and folders in a systematic way. Estimate the time required to complete each project. Have your own turnaround time sheet for different kinds of projects and number of pages. Maintain an excel sheet to keep track of projects and timelines. This sheet must have client name, project name, number of pages, date of initiation, projected date of completion, first-cut, final cut, date of closure, and remuneration status. Use a planner to spread your projects and at any point you should be able to judge the time required to complete the existing project and schedule future projects. As far as possible, your planner should be practical. Do not take more projects than what you can handle. Clients are always in a hurry. Do not underestimate the time required to complete a project. If you are planning to outsource your work, ensure that quality and timelines are never compromised. Keep your clients informed about the timelines.

Before accepting a project, check for project feasibility. Do not hesitate to ask for the references from clients. Once you accept a project, send a schedule depicting your work progress (understanding the project requirement, collecting references, developing an outline, writing, copyediting, and final draft). Always keep your references in order, so that you can provide them to the clients, if required. Try to establish contacts with people who have access to full- text article.

39.4 Writing

Understand the client needs and the topic given. Search for appropriate references. Read and understand the references. Conceptualize a content/outline that is appropriate for the topic. Even before actually writing, it is very important to keep in mind the client's specifications on the project.

- **Length of article:** Number of pages/ Number of words/Number of characters.
- **Line spacing:** Single, double or standard multiple (1.15) spacing
- **Font type and size:** Times New Roman (12 pt) or Calibri (11)
- **Images/graphs/tables:** Check if the graphs and tables have to be created in a Word file or copy-pasted as an image from the source pdf. Images should be suggestive and keep the client informed about the copyright of images. Not all images are free. Provide the URL so that, if needed, your client would be able to buy the image. If you create graphs from the data given, then you can charge for the graph developed and it can be considered as a part of the content developed. Tables that are created or typed can be considered as a part of the text.

39.5 Copyediting

You could either do the copyediting yourself or send the file to your copyeditor along with the reference pack. Do not review your article immediately; review it after a couple of hours, or a day before you send the document. Create your own checklist for reviewing. You can use the same checklist that we have provided in the chapter 16: Revision. Do a spell check to eliminate glaring spell errors.

39.6 Accounts

Confirm the project with terms and conditions that include your payment details. Immediately after the submission of the project, send your invoice. By default, most payments are made only after the approval of the client. Generally, a 30-day period is expected to receive payment for an article. Maintain a proper account of the projects, its actual cost, and your charges along with the date of initiation and date of delivery. Keep track of the pending payments. You may have to make multiple follow-ups to get payments. Don't hesitate to call or remind your client about pending payment.

39.7 How to Charge your Clients

You should calculate the total project cost based on various costs that you will incur.

1. Know the market rates.
2. Know the time required to complete the project
3. Know your investments (power, internet, stationary, computer, printer)

39.8 Timeline

Deliver the projects as agreed upon. Delivering projects on time will win further projects as it leaves the clients happy. You should refuse to take projects, which you cannot deliver within the timeline required by the client. Be professional in your approach. Never assume that you can ask for extra time after the project is initiated. Nevertheless, sometimes you can ask for extra time a couple of days before the set timeline, but never on the day the client is expecting your article to be delivered.

39.9 Quality

Make it your goal to deliver quality work. Your quality will be assessed by the references you use for writing the document, grammar, spelling mistakes, and style of writing. Acquiring good references will require knowledge, skills, and experience. It is mandatory to spell-check your document before sending it to the client. Avoid silly mistakes. Never make spelling mistakes in the title, heading, or subheadings; this will put off the client. Keep your references consistent. Make sure that abbreviations and acronyms are given according to the style prescribed by the client.

Practical Tips

Working as a freelancer gives flexibility to work and avoid commuting. Nevertheless, it requires a lot of discipline in bringing professionalism into freelance work. Distractions with domestic work, friends and families will be challenging. Remember and keep the following things in mind to become a successful and a professional freelancer.

Do's
• Give a professional touch to your work
• Have a separate work area that simulates an office atmosphere
• Keep your office space clean and tidy
• Maintain a regular work-hours or work-days
• Dress properly as you would go for work
• Maintain a work schedule (time table) on project basis
• Project your project timelines with a day as buffer
• Make adequate time for writing
• Make sure you work for at least 2 h at a stretch
• Concentrate on your work when writing
• Make list of things (at least 5) that you need to do for the day
• If possible, keep a separate telephone or mobile for work
• Take breaks in between work
• Keep your family and friends informed about your work-days or work-hours
• Maintain a log book of hours spent for each project
• Eat your proper meals
• Catch with your ex-colleagues when you need to break away from midday nap
• Speak to clients beyond work
• Establish a network
• Invest time and money in courses that can add-value to your profession
• Take up different kinds of medical writing and different types of projects for different audiences
• Know your area of expertise.

Dont's
• Do not frequently jumble household work and writing
• Do not work in your home dress (night suits)
• Do not compromise on sleep/family time/eating time
• Do not postpone your work to the last minute
• Do not underestimate the time required
• Do not miss project timelines
• Avoid too many activities in a day
• Do not fail to call other freelancers or your mentor in case of any doubts
• Do not entertain friends and relatives during your work hours
• Do not work while viewing television or listening to music
• Don't just speak to your clients, at times, have a video chat and establish connectivity

Chapter - 40

Copyediting

Almost 20% of medical writers also work as copyeditors. Some of you may have to check/review articles written by your colleagues/juniors as you climb up in the hierarchy. Therefore, you need to know about copyediting. As a copyeditor, you should ensure that the document is error-free and in accordance with the in-house style. You should also understand that copyediting and proofreading are not the same. Copyediting involves grammar corrections; maintaining consistency (e.g., for abbreviations); conformation to in-house/client style guides; coherence in content flow; cross checking facts with cited references; checking for fair use of references (making sure copyright issues are not violated); and eliminating illogical errors. Proofreading involves checking a document against the original for any errors of omission or commission. Proofreaders usually check the formatted/designed documents with the original for any typographical errors; omission of words/paragraphs; introduction of words/paragraphs; and accuracy of the formatted tables and graphs. However, medicomarketing companies cannot usually afford to hire two different people for copyediting and proof reading. Most of the time, copyeditors are required to perform the job of a proofreaders' too! To maintain standards, it is better if you learn to use the copyeditor's marks, which refer to the desired changes suggested by the copyeditor.

Conventionally copyediting has three different levels: Light, medium, and heavy copyediting. It is rather important to know how each level is different from each other. You can refer to any of the standard books on copyediting for knowing the different levels. In our set-up, copyeditors usually do a light copyediting along with few additional features from medium and heavy copyediting.

40.1 Light Editing

Mechanical Editing; Conforming to the in-house style guides; taking care of capitalizations, abbreviations, spellings, punctuations and hyphenation; and maintaining consistency in lists.

Correlations: Querying any misrepresentation of facts or data; cross-checking facts with references provided; querying any gap in the logical flow of content; checking and correcting citations of figures and tables in the document; cross-checking the contents page with the inside content; checking for reference order; checking the serial numbers of tables and figures; and checking table and figure footnotes.

Language Editing: Grammar and syntax corrections; querying lengthy, wordy, or convoluted paragraphs; and querying any part of the content/idea/concept that is not clear.

40.2 Medium Editing Involves

Mechanical Editing: Conforming to the in-house style guides; taking care of capitalizations, abbreviations, spelling, punctuations and hyphenation; maintaining consistency in lists.

Correlations: Quering any misrepresentation of facts or data; checking and correcting citations of figures and tables in the document; cross-checking the contents page with the inside content; serial referencing; serial numbering of tables and figures; and checking table and figure footnotes.

Language Editing: Grammar and syntax corrections; changing the voice of the sentence; querying lengthy, wordy or convoluted paragraphs and giving suggestions for changes; querying any part of the content/idea/concept that is not clear, and offering suggestions to the writer to give additional information, if required.

40.3 Heavy Copyediting Involves

Mechanical Editing: Conforming to the in-house style guides; taking care of capitalizations, abbreviations, spelling, punctuations and hyphenation; maintaining consistency in lists.

Copy Editing and Proofreading Symbols

Symbol	Meaning	Example
ℰ	Delete	Remove the ~~end~~ fitting.
◠	Close up	The tolerances are with in the range.
ℰ	Delete and close up	Del~~e~~te and close up the gap.
∧	Insert	The box is ∧inserted correctly. *not*
#	Space	The#procedure is incorrect.
∿	Transpose	Remove the fitting end.
/ or lc	Lower case	The Engineer and manager agreed.
≡	Capitalize	A representative of <u>nasa</u> was present.
╱	Capitalize first letter and lower case remainder	/GARRETT/PRODUCTS are great.
stet	Let stand	Remove the ~~battery~~ cables. *stet*
¶	New paragraph	The box is full.¶The meeting will be on Thursday.
no ¶	Remove paragraph break	The meeting will be on Thursday. ¶ *no* All members must attend.
⭢	Move to a new position	All members attended who were new.

Copy Editing and Proofreading Symbols...contd

Symbol	Meaning	Example
⌐	Move left	⌐Remove the faulty part.
⌐	Flush left	⌐Move left.
⌐	Flush right	⌐Move right.
⌐	Move right	⌐Remove the faulty part.
⌐ ⌐	Center	⌐Table 4-1⌐
⌐	Raise	16_2
⌐	Lower	16^2
∧	Superscript	162
∨	Subscript	162
⊙	Period	Rewrite the procedure. Then complete the tasks.
∨	Apostrophe or single quote	The company's policies were rewritten.
∧	Semicolon	He left; however, he returned later.
∧	Colon	There were three items: nuts, bolts, and screws.
∧	Comma	Apply pressure to the first, second, and third bolts.
-|	Hyphen	A valuable by-product was created.

Copy Editing and Proofreading Symbols...*contd*

Symbol	Meaning	Example
⬭ *sp*	Spell out	The ⬭info⬭ was incorrect. *sp*
◯	Abbreviate	The part was ⬭twelve⬭ ⬭feet⬭ long.
‖ or =	Align	Personnel Facilities ‖ Equipment
_____	Underscore	The part was listed under <u>Electrical</u>.
⁓	Run in with previous line	He rewrote the pages) (and went home.
⊥ /\/\	Em dash	It was the beginning so I thought. /\/\
⊥ /\/	En dash	The value is 120⊥408. /\/
⬭*ital*⬭	Set in italics	The book was titled <u>Technical Writing Styles</u>. ⬭*ital*⬭
⬭*bf*⬭	Set in bold	This is the <u>only</u> time we can offer this price. ⬭*bf*⬭
⬭*wf*⬭	Wrong font	This is the <u>**first step in the procedure**</u>. ⬭*wf*⬭
⬭*sm cap*⬭ =	Set in small caps	Set the <u>MFG REGISTER</u> to zero. ⬭*sm cap*⬭

Correlations: Verifying the incorrect facts or data and revising the content; querying any misrepresentation of facts or data; checking and correcting citations of figures and tables in the document; cross-checking the contents page with the inside content; serial referencing; serial numbering of tables and figures; and checking table and figure footnotes.

Language Editing: Grammar and syntax corrections; changing the voice of the sentence, if required; rewriting lengthy, wordy or convoluted sentences/paragraphs; querying any part of the content/idea/concept that is not clear and offering suggestions to the writer to give additional information, if required.

Ten Rules of Proof Reading

1. Never proofread your own copy.
2. Read everything in the copy straight through from the beginning to end.
3. Read copy backward to catch spelling errors.
4. Read pages out of order.
5. Have proofreaders initial the copy they check.
6. Have someone read numbers while you check hardcopy.
7. Take short breaks so you can concentrate more clearly.
8. List errors you spot over a month.
9. Alter your routine.
10. Make your marks legible and understandable.

Chapter - 41

Writing a Proposal

A proposal is a document used to persuade a customer to buy something. It offers a solution to a problem or a course of action in response to a need. It also indicates why you are the right person to conduct the project! A proposal contains following:

- Cover letter
- Details about the medicomarketing communication company
- Background on the need for the proposed project
- Description of the proposed project
- Benefits of the proposed project
- Specifications/Costs
- Schedule
- Terms and conditions

You may not need all of these elements, and some of them can be combined into single sentences. The proposal ought to be succinct and should not be verbose.

The cover letter states the topic, purpose of the proposal, and an overview of the contents. It should be concise. Nowadays, an email itself can serve as a cover letter. In addition to the email, you can write a formal cover letter, if required.

If you are writing a proposal on behalf of a medicomarketing communication company, it is important to introduce the company to the client. 'About the company' is like a 'mini-resume' of the company. Here you will justify the strength and capability of your team. It will include, the qualifications and credibility of the delivery team, lists of the work experience, similar projects completed, staff education, and experience that show familiarity with the project.

The sales team could help you understand the marketing needs of the client. In the background section, you have to state the problem, describes the factors that have contributed to the problem, and propose what can be done. Basically, show that you understand the problem!

Describe the finished product of the proposed project. Choose a title that conveys information about your project. Provide an outline of what you propose to write. Then list down the benefits of distributing such literature. The benefits are the heart and soul of a proposal. They acts as an argument in favor of approving the project.

The specifications to be given include

- Number of pages
- Size
- Color
- Frequency
- Number of issues.

Another important part of the proposal is schedule. It gives information on not only the projected completion date but also key milestones for the project. The timeline serves as a delivery progress report. If you cannot propose specific dates, give an approximate number of days required for each phase of the project.

Terms and conditions usually contain credit period, penalty clause, and tax liabilities.

41.1   Requisites of Proposal Writing

In a medicomarketing communications company, business development executives and medical writers write the proposal. Before writing the proposal, you should seek answers to the following questions:

- What do you know about client's requirement?
- What are your client's goals?
- What kind of projects does your sponsor support?
- What information does your client require?
- What format does your client expect?

The medical writer is the right person to suggest the input and topics. It is easy to suggest different types of inputs: booklets, brochures, newsletters, patient education, etc. However, what goes into the input is important. You have to think like a marketing manager. You should know treatment options and the unique selling points (USP) of each option. You are going to convert the available literary evidence into a marketing input. Suggest a promotion plan than a single input. You can suggest topics for series of booklets or brochures or newsletters based on the following:

- Different indications
- USP of the molecule
- Comparative studies
- Different patient profiles

You may need to describe the content for each topic. Other than suggesting topics, you may have to suggest interesting names for the newsletter and names for different sections in the newsletter. You have to be creative and innovative to suggest interesting titles.

A good presentation cannot substitute a weak idea; however, the greatest idea, presented ineffectively, would often fail! A good proposal is not the end, it is the beginning; it needs good execution. Sometimes, proposals fail due to various reasons:

- Topic unrelated to client's requirement and goal
- Unclear problem, objectives, or project plan lack of clarity about the need
- Lack of focus, overly ambitious
- Benefits of the project not clear
- Been done before, lacks novelty
- Cost
- Carelessness (typographical errors, misspelling, and omitted words) is usually perceived as a harbinger of future careless work on the project

Chapter - 42

Medical Writer as a Manager

A medical writer has to move up the career ladder to become a team lead/manager/head. As one moves up the career ladder, the roles and responsibilities also vary. Many times, writers are not equipped to become good managers; nevertheless, if one understands the roles and responsibilities of the post/designation, it is easy to manage a team of writers and facilitate smooth workflow. A manager's responsibilities include:

- Developing and maintaining a cordial relationship with co-workers
  - ➤ provide all kinds of professional and work support to the team
  - ➤ be a mentor/guide
  - ➤ engage in effective team building strategies
  - ➤ manage conflicts

- Getting and giving information
  - ➤ Keep the team informed about the project or project changes or change in management policies.
  - ➤ As and when need arises, clarify the team members' doubts/apprehensions about projects/issues
  - ➤ From time to time, monitor project progress within the team to avoid last minute hiccups

- Making decisions
  - ➤ Either plan and organize the work for the team or involve the team in planning and organizing project delivery
  - ➤ Be available to solve problems for the team
  - ➤ Delegate work to the team members according to their strengths and weaknesses

- Influencing people
  - ➢ Be an inspiration to the team and keep them motivated to perform better
  - ➢ Never fail to recognize any important contribution made by the team members towards the betterment of the company
  - ➢ Find different ways to reward the deserving members of the team

An extraordinary manager is one who makes things happen, despite adversities. They get extraordinary results from ordinary people. As most medical writers are from pharmacy, medical, or life science background, we do not study management as a subject. In addition, most medical writers are promoted as managers/team lead without proper training or preparation. Any medical writer wanting to scale up the career ladder should be ready for some introspection. He/she must always keep the following in check:

- Know your strengths and weakness
- Develop skills that you are lacking
- Compensate for your weaknesses by selecting people with complementary skills and delegate work

Few other important challenges faced by a manager include:

- Interviewing
- Training
- Motivating
- Retaining good talent
- Doing performance appraisal

42.1   Selecting and Retaining Good Talent

One rotten apple in a basket spoils the whole basket. It is very important to select the right candidate for the job. Hiring a wrong person can affect the growth and reputation of the organization. They can affect the morale and confidence of colleagues and clients. It also increases attrition. Selecting a right candidate is tough. Even Chief Executive Officers (CEOs) make mistakes while selecting people. My success rate for selecting good writers was 40%. Never be in a hurry to fill a vacancy. If you do not find the right candidate, it is better to leave a post vacant than to hire someone who can negatively affect your organization.

Hiring medical writers usually goes through 2-3 stages. Besides the personal interview, the candidate has to complete a written assignment consisting of a review article (3-4 pages), medical news, and an essay (each not more than one page). There might be two rounds of personal interview, one before the assignment and the other after the assignment. All three stages are crucial for both the interviewee and the interviewer.

I have tried to recruit people through human resource consultants, job portals, advertisements, personal contacts, campus recruitment, and employee referrals. No method is fool proof. Do everything possible to get a good candidate.

Do your homework before interviewing. Always fix an appointment for the interview and remember it! Be ready for the interview before the candidate arrives. Read his/her resume, make a list of questions to ask, and be prepared to explain about your company and the job profile. If you cannot be present for the interview, delegate it to someone and inform accordingly. A good performance during personal interview with the candidate does not guarantee his performance at work; nevertheless, by asking the right question, you can avoid selecting a bad candidate. A person may answer some tough questions very well but may fail to write well. Ask questions to assess the follow:

- Candidate's experience against job requirement
- Communication skills
- Team work
- Importance of quality
- Orientation towards result
- Functional expertise
- Flexibility Client focus
- "Can do" attitude
- Career plan
- Salary expectations

Do not ask a question that allows someone to give 'text book' answers. Do not ask negative questions like "What are your weaknesses?" or "Tell me about your failures". Frame the same questions differently to get the right answers. Ask questions specific to assignments done, clients handled (to know how the candidate performed his previous work in his earlier company), what problems he faced, how he handled them, and what the results were. You do not have to ask 101 questions to assess him/her; even 5-6 questions may give you a fair idea about the person. Also, be open to your intuition/gut feeling about the candidate (if your intuition works well for you).

If you come across an outstanding candidate, do not procrastinate. Do not wait for the next round of interview. Be quick to grab them. At the same time, do not commit if you do not have the authority to hire. If someone else has to do the next round of interview, try to fix it as quickly as possible (if possible, at that moment).

Be positive about your company and the job profile. Most of the time, you have to 'sell' the job. At least for medical writers, it is required. I had to sell the job every time. Candidates did not know about medical writing as a full-time profession. I had to learn about the profession thoroughly to sell the job (the result of that is the book you are reading!). I would explain to the candidate, like a story, about my company, the need for medical marketing communication, types of articles, product life cycle, typical project flow, career path, what differentiates us from competitors, opportunity for growth etc. Once the interview is over, intimate the candidate about the process. Inform positive or negative results, when to expect the next call etc. Send them the offer letter, if selected.

42.2 Induction/Orientation

Make every effort to make the new employee feel that he has joined the best place to work on the first day. Even before an employee joins, identify his/her place at the office, keep it ready with a computer, stationery, phone etc. Many atimes, the manager turns up later than the new employee and they would have to wait in the reception. Avoid such awkward situations for the new employee. They cannot be staring at people walking around sitting in the reception. Introduce the new employee to everyone. Announce, through mail, to other offices about the new employee, who has joined. Show the new employee the cafeteria, toilets, etc (maybe silly, but think of yourself searching for the toilet in a new place). It is good to ask the new employee to accompany you for coffee and lunch for a day or have a person to chaperon him/her. Once the formal introduction is complete, begin orientation to the job. Provide them the standard operating procedures (SOPs) or work manual

42.3 Retaining Good Talent

Attrition costs time and money. You would have spent time and energy to train an employee. If someone with good talent and attitude wants to quit the company, it may signal a problem with you or the system or organization. Many a times, people leave because of other people, not for money or position. Take a proactive approach to avoid losing good talent. Be alert to signs that signal that an employee is demotivated. Watch for these signs:

- Drop in productivity
- Increased absenteeism
- No involvement in work
- Discussions about employees who left
- Isolation from other employees
- Irritability
- Talk about pressure, stress

Do not ignore such signals. Talk to them; listen to them. Offer them solutions to the problems and convert the promise into actions. Do not allow them to remind you about the promise you made. Sometimes you may not be able to identify an employee wanting to leave and take preventive action. People do resign, but not everything is over. Talk to them quickly. Ask them about the reasons for resignation, any new offer they are considering, etc. Try to do whatever you can to retain them. Nevertheless, do not make counter offers with more money. Those who want to leave for more money will leave after taking the counter-offer. They may use your counter-offer to negotiate with the new employer. Besides, other employees may also use the same technique to get more money. Sometimes, counter-offers may backfire. Employees may think that you should have paid earlier and that you have no budget constraints when a situation arises.

In any company, you will find 3 categories of employees, depending on performance and attitude.

1. Outstanding performers with negative opinions about the company and colleagues (negative attitude)
2. Average performers with positive opinions
3. Non-performers with positive or negative opinions

Some employees should be dismissed as soon as possible. An outstanding performer with negative attitude is like a rotten apple. Even though he is good at work, he may influence others with his negative attitude. An average performer with positive attitude is better than an outstanding performer with negative attitude. A nonperformer should anyway be dismissed.

42.4   Understand What People want from Work

Although everybody wants money from work, it is not everything. Nobody thinks about money every day while working. They will think about money only when they do not get their salary on time or a good increment. They want many other things from the job. Many researchers have conducted studies to find out what people want from work.

Everyone works for money. Everybody wants money for food, shelter, clothing, security, family needs, etc. People are self-motivated to work for survival needs. Beyond survival needs, there are a lot other things that people expect from work.

- Sense of achievement
- Appreciation/recognition
- Interesting/challenging work
- Responsibility
- Position and promotion
- Supervision/leadership
- Good working conditions
- Social status

Not everybody needs all of the above. The needs of each person are different. Identify the individual needs of the members of your team and try to meet them. Here are a few things you can do to meet their needs and motivate them.

42.5   Question the Purpose of Work

Ask your employees

- Why do they work?
- For whom do they work?

- Who pays their salary?
- What should they do for them?

Everybody works for money and other needs as discussed earlier. Explain the purpose of working for clients, who indirectly pay the employees' salaries. Therefore, it is the responsibility of each of the team members to meet the clients' needs and expectations. Our clients expect us to deliver quality products on time. If we deliver quality products according to their timeline, we are helping them succeed. They feel happy and we get more business. If we get more business, we achieve our targets. The management or the shareholders of the company do not keep all the money for themselves. They share it with the employees.

42.6 Show the Bigger Picture

Another way to inspire people is to show how the business works. Everybody needs to know about how the business works beyond his or her job to succeed. Explain each process involved in the business and organization. Explain the importance of their role. Use a flow chart or algorithm to explain the flow of work. Explain how a company makes money and how each person can contribute to earn more money. It helps them have an overview of the business. In addition, share monthly, quarterly, and annual results, projects, and success stories; send a thank you note for helping to achieve targets.

42.7 Discuss Competition

Knowing about competitors helps the team, the company understand where the company stands in the market, and how it is doing compared to them. It is another way of showing the big picture of the business. Competition generates excitement and enthusiasm among the team to do better. Make a presentation on your competitors to show their 'strengths, weaknesses, opportunities, and threats' and discuss on these lines.

- Who are they?
- What is their turnover/revenue?
- What is their market share?
- Who are their clients?
- Who are the key people?
- What types of products/services do they offer?

- How are they different from our company?
- What do clients think about them and us?
- What is the process they follow to execute projects?

Do not highlight only the negative points of competitors. Use their strengths to learn and adopt good things from them. Try to collect samples of projects done by the competitor and share them with others. Share examples of winning a project against a competitor.

- How and why did we win over our competitors?
- Why did we lose projects to our competitors?
- How should we handle them?

42.8   Ask for New Ideas

The world is changing very fast. There will be new competitors, new technologies, and new models/products every day. To survive in the changing environment, we need new ideas. They need not come only from top management. Inspire creative thinking among employees by asking them to suggest new ideas and models for the company. Some of them may not work immediately, however having a bank of ideas is good to propose options to the clients. They will be useful at some point or other. Sometimes, one idea or theme gets you another project.

42.9   You get What you Ask for Challenge Them

Another important point is to set and raise the standards of performance. Tell your team about your expectations. You will get what you ask for. If the performance standards you set are low, they will meet them. If you set higher standards, they will try to meet them. Make the work challenging. Set goals beyond the perceived limits, so that everybody stretches beyond their abilities. Also set rewards for achieving goals, but do not promise rewards if you do not have the authority.

42.10   Appreciate Good Work

Whenever you find good points or good work done by others, appreciate it. People feel happy to be appreciated. Send an appreciation mail for achieving the goals or publically display achievements on the notice board. This will increase the visibility of employees or groups. Showcasing success makes people feel proud.

42.11 Create a Cool Environment

I always thought we are in a serious business and fun dilutes the seriousness, but fun helps connect with people faster. It makes work more enjoyable. Introduce some humor during training; this helps people learn faster. Fun also makes people overcome inhibitions. At the same time too much of fun will disturb the work. Ensure that humor does not hurt others. Protect people's dignity and self-respect all the time.

42.12 Share Tips/Examples

Have informal meetings to share experiences/tips related to work. Everybody can collect good articles and discuss good points. They can also share new resources that they found.

42.13 Train Them

A job becomes burden if an employee does not have right skills. Help them to acquire skills so that work becomes pleasure for them. Training is my passion. I have conducted training sessions on different aspects of our business. I make presentations whenever I come across topics relevant to medical communication. I have conducted training on all the topics discussed in this book. In fact, I seek external trainers to give their expertise and impart training to my team. It may be as simple as a refresher course in English.

Chapter - 43

Writer's Block

There comes a time in every writer's life, when it becomes difficult to continue writing, and suddenly there is a prolonged slump in work productivity. During this time, the writer suffers from temporary loss of ability to begin or continue writing, usually due to lack of inspiration or creativity. Such phase is called writer's block. Writer's block is a common phenomenon with not only medical writing, but also with other creative writing streams. Every writer should know what can be done when it occurs, and what steps can be taken to prevent it.

43.1   What Causes Writer's Block

- Self-consciousness about your writing: Writer's block happens because of a "right brain-left brain" conflict. The right or creative side of the brain wants to write. This induces the left or analytical side of the brain to anticipate all the problems that this action could lead to, causing it to go into "overdrive" and inhibit the ability to write.

- **Anxiety and stress:** Many things like deadlines and difficult topics can cause anxiety and stress. It encourages procrastination, causing confusion and totally freezing the thought processes.

- Perfectionism can cause writer's block as it leads to anxiety. It is important to remember that one can always revise the content and the first draft need not be perfect.

- Lack of planning can often be a cause of block when a writer does not know how to go forward. You may be attempting to write without doing any preliminary work such as reading, understanding, brainstorming, or planning. It is important that you have some idea as to what data goes into each of the sections.

- Writer's block can happen due to physical stress, lack of sleep, depression, and bad health.

- Adverse working environments that cause continuous disturbances while writing (noisy environment, talkative colleagues, or frequent visitors)

- **Excuses:** We also try to find hundreds of excuses to postpone writing an article.

43.2   What can you do to Overcome Writer's Block?

What you can do to overcome writer's block depends on the cause. First, try to identify the cause. Each of the above discussed causes can be overcome. First, reassure yourself that this problem is temporary and can be successfully resolved with time, patience, and appropriate remediation.

- **Set realistic goals:** If your left brain is stopping you from writing by thinking about the problems, set your expectations right. You may be setting unrealistic expectations for yourself. Either you want to write huge amounts in a single sitting or you want to write a perfect document the first time. Both are wrong. Split the articles into sections and write one part of the article at one go. Do not try to be a perfectionist in the first draft. Challenge negative thoughts about your skill or ability to write.

- Most of the time, writer's block among medicomarketing writers is because of impossible deadlines. Do not think about the deadline too much. Continue to write section by section in a qualitative manner. Thinking about the deadline will only worsen the situation than improving it.

- Another major reason for writer's block is beginning to write without clarity about the topic. You should try to read and understand the topic. Discuss/brainstorm with others before beginning to write. Explain what you want to write. It helps you understand the topic better. Review the references you have collected and, if necessary, reorganize the references and notes. Write a basic outline of the article to keep the story on track.

- **Improve working conditions:** If you are not able to write because of noise or disturbances by your colleagues, talk to them about the disturbance. Request them to not disturb you. If your table, chair, or computer is hindering your writing, see what you can do to improve the comfort. Fix a deadline to write, regardless of the quality of the output. Do not try to write a perfect article in first attempt itself.

- If you have to do too many different things at a time, you may end up completing none of them. Plan your work. Prioritize the work you have and do one work at a time.

- Occasionally, none of these suggestions works. You may simply need a break. Turn off the computer and call it a day. Go for a walk. Listen to music. Seek out a friend and share a few jokes. Laugh at yourself. Lighten up. Then the next day, try again. By then things might have unconsciously worked themselves out.

- The last option is to resign yourself to the fact that you have to write for your bread and butter.

43.3   How can you Prevent Writer's Block?

- The key to prevention is to minimize anxiety about writing, and the best way to do this is by starting early.

- Most people collect more data than they need to write. Faced with the sheer volume of data, you can easily get lost if you have not written an outline or planned your article. Collect whatever is necessary.

- Cultivate an interest in writing. Read books on medical writing and writing in general. Visit relevant online sites on the Internet and sign up for a workshop or conference that offers courses in medical writing.

Chapter - 44

Performance Appraisal

Performance appraisal is a feedback given to employees to improve employee performance. However, for most managers and employees, performance appraisal is a pain. Many performance reviews do more harm than good. They often do not help the manager-employee relationship, but strains the relationship. At times, the morale of the employee is diminished. Nevertheless, if you treat an employee as responsible, intelligent, important members of the organization, performance appraisals will be beneficial. The objectives of performance appraisals are:

- To evaluate each employee's performance against previously set goals

- To provide a forum for open discussion of an employee's performance against expectations

- To improve the employee's performance through constructive feedback and the setting of development plans

- To assist in effective salary revision

- To know the needs of training

Explain the objective of the appraisal beforehand so that the employee understands the need and is prepared for the interview.

To assess the performance of an individual, you should identify and define the performance categories and parameters used.

44.1   Performance Categories

An important part of the appraisal is the performance categories used to assess performance. The categories for appraisal and their definitions are given below:

| Parameters | Incorrigible | Poor | Satisfactory | Good | Excellent |
	1	2	3	4	5
Business understanding					
About medical marketing communication					
About the pharma industry					
Ability to understand the client's requirement/ understanding the brief					
Skill and knowledge					
Technical knowledge					
Resourcing ability					
Optimizing the search					
Effective use of keywords					
Turnaround time					
Ability to read and understand					
Understanding					
Interpreting data					
Analyzing the study					
Summarizing					
Turnaround time					

Parameters	Incorrigible 1	Poor 2	Satisfactory 3	Good 4	Excellent 5
Ability to write					
Uniformity/Consistency					
Grammar					
Pre-checking of documents					
Mistakes/Revisions required					
Tables/Figures/Captions					
Variety in articles					
Turnaround time					
Project completion					
Adherence to timelines					
Responsibility of completing					
Quality of the article submitted					
Process					
Understanding					
Adherence					

Parameters	Incorrigible 1	Poor 2	Satisfactory 3	Good 4	Excellent 5
Communication					
Language skills					
Email etiquette					
Communication with HOD					
Communication with team lead					
Communication with team members					
Management skills					
Activity management					
Coordination within the team					
Coordination with designers					
Coordination with marketing					
Coordination with client					
Crisis management/pressure handling					
Follow-up of projects					

Parameters	Incorrigible	Poor	Satisfactory	Good	Excellent
	1	2	3	4	5
Soft skills					
Ability to learn					
Involvement in training/Presentations made					
Discipline					
Attendance					
Health					
Overall assessment (Tick appropriate head)	Unsatis-factory	Need to improve	Meets	Meets Plus	Exceeds

Excellent: Consistently exceeds the established performance measures and contributes beyond job requirements

Good: Consistently meets the established performance measures and frequently exceeds those in multiple areas or ways

Satisfactory: Consistently meets the established performance measures

Needs development: Occasionally meets the established performance measures.

Unsatisfactory: Does not meet the established performance measures

44.2 Parameters

The following parameters are particular to medical writers. As parameters used for assessment are subjective, it is better to discuss them before the appraisal interview.

44.3 Few Things to Keep in Mind

- Do performance appraisals long before salary increment time
- If you feel someone is being unfairly compensated, discuss this with management and human resources.
- Be careful not to make any promises you won't be able to keep.
- Keep another person while doing appraisal.
- Do periodic appraisals instead of one annual appraisal.